WHAT YOU NEED TO KNOW ABOUT YOUR MORAL HEALTH

Andre Antao

DEDICATION

In memory of my father,

Zacharias 1929-1989.

CONTENTS

INTRODUCTION

The world is currently experiencing significant upheaval. We are navigating through challenging and demanding circumstances. There is a prevailing sense of uncertainty regarding the future of humanity and our planet. Globally, it is evident that we live in an environment fraught with danger. Evildoing resembles a pandemic in our world, and there appears to be no remedy for the virus that fuels evil actions. The decline of moral standards in the postmodern era is a reflection of humanity's overall moral health.

In our society, virtues are often poorly recognized and undervalued. The aesthetics of human life is lost to the human sense. We have strayed from the noble ideals once pursued, such as leaving a legacy of admirable deeds, noble actions, and virtuous living. Conversely, we often lack clarity, as well as the willingness and courage to recognize evil for what it truly is.

Machiavellian tendencies dominate modern life, with Machiavellianism shaping how life feels—chaotic and diabolically complex. For most people, if not everyone, there is no better way to live. The so-called "high Machs" hold uncontested influence. This has led many to believe that their inhumane acts and evil deeds are trivial. Victims harmed by powerful entities, such as corporations and political institutions, often fail to receive proper justice. Daily life is usually marred by vicious rudeness, malicious vindictiveness, and savage brutality.

In the postmodern world, technological advancements have a significant impact on the concept of human identity. Advances in technology often overshadow innate human qualities, especially spiritual and moral dimensions. There is a noticeable tendency to overlook the metaphysical aspects of human existence today. As a result, the fabric of human life is constructed on an unstable moral base rooted in sensuality, irrationality, and dishonesty. This separation diminishes higher-level personhood and weakens the view of a complete self defined by integrity, character, virtue, principles, nobility, honor, and noble attitudes—elements that embody the profound richness of human essence.

Every day, we fall short in the difficult work required to develop the higher-level personhood of a holistic self. Our daily lives are not rooted in higher ideals and goals. We live in denial of the existential truth and reality of human existence. We judge one another based on traditional morality and superficial socio-cultural standards. We view moral well-being through the lens of conventional morality, which not only results in judgments, blame, and condemnation of others but also causes us to avoid personal and social responsibility, resist self-improvement, and deny the fundamental aspects of human reality and life. We ignore experiences of moral sickness within ourselves, others, and society.

Most people do not see moral health as part of overall well-being. When considering each other's moral welfare, the focus is mainly on adherence to conventional morality rather than on moral health. Attention is often placed on moral standards rather than moral health. There is a tendency to overlook the impact of the moral self on moral health. Additionally, when evaluating the moral self, it is based on moral standards, not higher-order personhood or psychosocial maturity. The link between the moral self, moral health, and the global moral environment is often ignored. As a result, our view of life's purpose and meaning is usually centered on a moral self that is either rigid or undeveloped, and ineffective or irrelevant.

We do not see moral disease as a health issue. The widespread evil of our time and people's harmful tendencies are not considered part of moral health. We often rely on court cases and legal punishments to address serious moral and ethical issues, rather than focusing on developing a higher level of personhood and holistic selfhood. Our education systems often fail to incorporate the cultivation of the moral self and the skills necessary to promote moral health.

The moral self of an individual is crucial to their overall moral well-being, which in turn influences the collective moral state of society, thereby shaping the moral environment globally. Our daily thoughts, feelings, and actions in the moral sphere reflect our moral self, which is brought to life. Low levels of moral health in individuals indicate a weak, distorted, or harmful moral self, which in turn affects the moral welfare of society. People are no longer aiming to immortalize their lives through good deeds, virtues, and noble service to the common good.

The weak, rigid, and malignant moral self that shapes people's lifestyles, priorities, and goals reflects a decline in the moral culture of our world. Every day, we encounter individuals who feign having a moral self to appear respectable socially, or whose actions are deeply harmful, threatening, and cause severe impacts on others. The media often reports on politicians, public figures, and celebrities who struggle to maintain their honorable public image. This demonstrates that society as a whole fails to succeed in fostering moral health as a crucial part of the "good life."

Today's global culture of materialism, individualism, and hedonism fosters a pathological self-centered attitude in living. People often find it challenging to be other-oriented, as they tend to focus mainly on themselves. It has resulted in people creating illusions about our identities, sometimes even trying to seem better than others. However, what appears conspicuous is also that many individuals' sense of self stems from insecurities and vulnerabilities. In modern society, people are like a bag of skin filled with illusions. Few are willing to accept that it is in everyday life that moral health and moral sickness develop.

Conventional morality focuses on social appearances and acceptability. We present an acceptable moral self to be considered decent and correct by society. We often display morality to avoid judgment, condemnation, and rejection. However, traditional morality, which supports social, legal, and religious institutions, is becoming less effective in the postmodern world at fostering moral health and often acts as a disruptive force in various areas of modern life.

Ordinarily, everyone upholds the role of moral conscience in being human. In literature, moral conscience is distinguished from people's moral consciousness. Scholars argue that growing in moral awareness is distinctly different from pursuing traditional moral ideals and principles. Conventional morality governs moral conscience but not moral awareness.

Those who scientifically study human consciousness describe the moral content of human consciousness as moral consciousness. People's moral awareness varies greatly from merely following moral standards. The pursuit of higher ideals and purposes, driven by a deeper understanding of moral complexities, demonstrates how moral consciousness manifests in individuals. It involves cognitive skills such as awareness, reasoning, sensory perception, and intuition, which help improve moral understanding and behavior more effectively than morality alone.

Throughout history, there are examples of individuals whose moral awareness has overridden their conscience, which led them to deceive, exploit, oppress, and take advantage of not just a few people but entire societies or nations for personal gain. When the focus shifts to cultivating moral health rather than merely avoiding moral violations, the limitations of traditional morality in promoting moral well-being and enhancing the moral welfare of society become apparent.

As a distinctly human phenomenon, moral consciousness enables a comprehensive awareness and understanding of the current moral situation. The moral phenomenon goes beyond space and time and cannot be confined to moral standards and ideals, as traditional morality suggests. The moral chaos in our world demonstrates that the prohibitions, inhibitions, and constraints of conventional morality are easily rationalized and justified in daily life.

What modern health sciences, especially neuroscience,

4

neurophysiology, psychiatry, and psychology, reveal is that the "moral brain" supports moral consciousness. Neuroscience has identified the brain regions responsible for moral awareness. Now, we are beginning to understand that human DNA contains a more profound moral sense, which helps us evaluate the quality of our daily choices and actions beyond traditional morality. This suggests that a person's decisions and actions may not only align with their conscience, shaped by abstract morality, but also stem from the moral consciousness that can sometimes be muted or less active.

Today, neuroscience research challenges the common belief that moral abilities depend on following traditional morality. Neuroscience provides evidence of a "moral brain" that is unique to humans, making humans distinctly moral beings within the animal kingdom and supporting moral well-being. Some scientists argue that the moral phenomenon is encoded in human DNA.

Few recognize the moral aspect of human nature as an integral part of human nature, and even fewer see moral health as a crucial component of overall health. However, modern health sciences show that moral health operates within the same cause-and-effect system as other natural elements. Health researchers emphasize that spiritual and moral aspects are essential human realities, and they also underscore that high levels of spiritual and moral health can enhance a person's overall health, encompassing physical, mental, and social aspects.

Health sciences show that moral health is the foundation for both positive and negative conditions affecting all other aspects of health. It becomes increasingly evident by the state of our chaotic and troubling world that low levels of moral health have serious consequences for the well-being of humanity and the planet. At the same time, these issues are personally experienced through adverse impacts on daily physical and mental health, as well as societal stability. Without individuals actively developing in human consciousness, the state of our personal and collective moral health will not improve.

This book considers moral health as part of the same cause-and-effect system that governs all of nature. It examines ideas of moral health and moral disease alongside scientific insights into human moral nature. By analyzing the moral climate of the time, the book helps readers understand the concept of moral disease as a health-related issue that impacts both individual and collective moral well-being. It offers a scientific perspective on moral health, distinct from abstract morality, and explores ways to promote and sustain moral health in these evolving times. It also demonstrates how moral health can contribute to creating a better world that we all want to live in.

The book emphasizes that moral health benefits individuals and also has a positive impact on society, humanity, and the planet. It points out that humanity's moral well-being is often overlooked when addressing global issues. To improve the moral climate worldwide, the focus should be on self-evolution and developing higher-order personhood rather than merely appearing moral by following traditional standards. The book encourages readers to see everyday actions not just in terms of good and evil or right and wrong, but as meaningful to overall moral health.

This book aims to highlight the serious consequences of poor moral health for both humanity and the planet. Ignoring our moral selves risks exacerbating global moral disease crises caused by the postmodern world culture, which is effectively eroding moral standards in human life. Neglecting moral health poses a threat to humanity's future. A glimpse into our human history reveals that major threats emerge when collective moral health declines.

MORAL DISEASE: A WORLDWIDE PUBLIC HEALTH CRISIS

Moral pain and suffering, often called "moral disease" in health literature, is an overlooked health issue. Today, both individuals and society are experiencing intense moral pain and suffering. We're failing to see it as a severe public health crisis worldwide.

More often than we like to admit, "moral disease" in both historical and modern times is the root cause of social issues, problems, and evils in society. The violence, crime, use of illegal drugs, social unrest and upheavals, communal tension, and unchecked hostility between individuals, groups, and nations are more a reflection of moral disease than anything else.

Moral disease is the oldest problem in human health and the deadliest in history. The global impact of moral disease today is reflected in the staggering statistics of suicides and homicides, overcrowded prisons and mental health clinics, the rise in gun violence, the widespread issue of illegal drug abuse, high overdose death rates, and much more.

Generally, we are less likely to see religious and political fanaticism in modern society as reflecting deeper issues of moral pain and suffering. Nor do we usually view the widespread abuses of political power and public office as signs of moral pain and suffering. Similarly, wars and genocides, racism and ethnic cleansing, the rise of terrorist groups and rebel factions, killings by suicide bombers, and mass murders — are they not also signs of moral disease? But aren't they, too?

In today's society, it often seems that the upper echelons, along with the famous and influential, remain untouched by moral corruption. However, a closer look reveals that many religious and political leaders, as well as social celebrities, use social status to hide deeper issues of moral pain and suffering. It is also often evident that the self-importance schemes of oligarchs, tycoons, moguls, tyrants, and despots show no clear purpose of moral integrity. The dominance of such individuals reflects character flaws more than personality disorders, as some believe. Their lifestyles, shameful behaviors, addiction problems, health issues, and even criminal activity do not hide the moral pain and suffering they experience.

Furthermore, and more importantly, geopolitical tensions and conflicts that threaten peace and harmony between nations are symptoms of a moral health crisis rather than solely political or economic problems. The conflicts caused by geopolitical disputes, socio-economic inequalities, racial tensions, and ideological extremism all point to a profound moral sickness in our world. These issues reveal that moral disease is a pervasive and unchecked pandemic in the postmodern world.

All inhumane and evil acts in our world demonstrate that moral illness is contagious. The dangerous, chaotic, and tumultuous nature of our times confirms the widespread presence of moral disease. The declining moral environment today underscores the significant amount of moral pain and suffering in human life. However, moral disease does not receive the attention it deserves and is often severely overlooked when addressing the challenges and problems humanity faces.

Moral disease is a health condition that is hard to define. Health experts point out that moral disease does not fit into physical, biochemical, psychological, or neurological categories.[1] However, there is also a viewpoint that the moral aspect of human nature remains a persistent issue in physical, mental, and social health. Health professionals contend that in many complex and unseen ways, moral pain and suffering cause serious harm to personal health and well-being, as well as to society and humanity's overall welfare.

The individual's experience of moral pain and suffering is the deep, often unseen psychological and emotional stress within their sense of self. Although it's frequently intangible, it manifests through psychological, emotional, and sometimes physical signs. It often results in uncontrolled self-sabotaging behaviors. Modern health sciences are beginning to uncover, through research, more complex internal issues that are usually overlooked, which exacerbate the challenges people encounter with their physical, mental, and social well-being.

Health sciences address the moral pain and suffering that underlie problematic behavioral issues, which negatively impact people's efforts in health promotion and disease prevention. Evidence in medical science indicates that moral pain and suffering can disrupt the body's homeostasis.[2] Mental health professionals argue that a person's sense of self-worth, resilience, and freedom are linked to both moral health and mental health. Social scientists point out that poor social health, which is significantly reflected by the gamut of societal problems, is rooted in the poor moral health of society. All social tensions, disorders, and issues stem from individuals' moral pain and suffering.

However, in modern times, one thing we often forget when thinking about health is that moral disease is a health-related condition. We tend to focus only on abstract morality, not on moral health and illness. Additionally, we overlook that the root of moral disease is the malignant moral self of personhood. The moral self can lead either to moral disease or moral health,

---

[1] Szasz, T. Diagnoses are not diseases. The Lancet; December 1991
[2] Quinter JL, et.al. Pain Medicine and Its Models: Helping or Hindering? Pain Medicine Vol. 9 Issue 7; 2008

and the moral self also influences all aspects of health.

The widespread presence of moral pain and suffering in our world suggests that people experience an intense sense of emptiness and a profound lack of meaning in life every day. This is the leading cause of non-organic mental health problems in society, more than any other aspect of postmodern life. Health researchers and scholars argue that many of modern society's issues—such as alcohol and drug abuse, violence and crime, racism and bigotry, as well as homicides and suicides—are direct or indirect results of moral disease rather than mental illness.[3]

The mental health crisis in modern society more strongly reflects people's deep moral pain and suffering than genetic or neurological conditions, as some in the scientific community often claim. While not all mental illness is caused by moral factors, many mental health issues on both personal and social levels are rooted in a destructive moral self of personhood.

Every day, behavioral anomalies, toxic and dysfunctional relationships, anxiety, depression, and other psycho-emotional conditions are interconnected effects of people's moral and mental health issues. When moral pain and suffering undermine one's self-worth, they create fertile ground for mental illness to develop. Usually, we find it hard to see that the moral self causes pathological psycho-emotional conditions and mental health problems. It is difficult for us to believe that the deviant and debased moral self of a person has anything to do with one's mental health or causes mental health issues in society.

People's psycho-emotional-social instability in society is more a sign of moral health decline than a mental health issue, as many suggest. It originates from the worldview of a self that harbors virulent moral values within individuals. Modern health science indicates that self-centeredness, permissiveness, and hedonism significantly contribute to the intense psycho-

---

[3] Hoover J., Atari M., et.al. Investigating the role of group-based morality in extreme behavioral expressions of prejudice. Nature Communications (vol. 12); (2021).

emotional stress people face, which can lead to mental health problems. Mental health experts believe that the pattern of mental health disorders reflects not only a lack of moral responsibility toward personal well-being but also neglect of the welfare of others.

The worldwide culture of our time, characterized by self-centeredness, causes more moral pain and suffering than we are willing to admit or recognize. The way we live in modern society clearly reflects a sense of pathological self-centeredness. Self-centeredness dominates people's values, attitudes, and priorities in daily life. Extreme self-centeredness leads to utilitarian individualism, which causes us to treat others as means to an end. It effectively destroys the cohesive sense of self and the other-orientedness of people.

Few will doubt that the epidemic of moral decadence in modern society stems from the widespread issue of utilitarian individualism. The belief that one's personal needs, desires, and freedom take precedence over the collective is a dominant force in today's human experience. Utilitarian individualism in modern society includes extreme self-centered behaviors that range from domination to exploitation.

Utilitarian individualism has led people to adopt a pleasure-seeking life orientation as the ultimate and unmatched approach to self-fulfillment. We poorly demonstrate the ability to recognize and validate the needs of others. We are reluctant to practice other-oriented thinking, attitudes, and values. We have misplaced the foundation of moral integrity and character, which should be based on respect for human dignity, tolerance, mutuality, social cohesion, and coexistence.

Utilitarian individualism shapes the virulent moral self of personhood, influencing how people perceive themselves and others as humans in modern society. Everyday biases, hostility, and violence reveal utilitarian individualism, exposing the psycho-emotional processes that affect our experience of humanity. The moral frameworks, ideological bonds, and toxic relationship patterns in modern society create confusion about what it means to be human.

11

Cultural critics argue that the outdated standards of abstract morality in postmodern times hinder or are ineffective in pursuing higher ideals, purposes, and the common good.

In modern society, the ethos of self-centeredness replaces the ethos of other-centeredness. It is clear in everyday life that people strive for self-fulfillment and happiness without considering that others have the same needs. This suggests that not everyone is willing to acknowledge or accept that the everyday pursuit of the "good life" must intersect with the moral self. It indicates that we lack the higher-order personhood that enables psychosocial maturity and effective relationship-building in modern society. We often overlook the fact that the ability for interdependence and human solidarity is a crucial pathway to building moral health or moral disease.

In modern society, people often overlook the fact that personal well-being also entails caring for others. However, the unseen effects of everyday selfish actions make us vulnerable to developing adverse inner psychic complexities, which often are the root cause of many psychological and emotional issues that may gradually lead to severe mental health problems.

When people passionately defend illogical social ideals that conflict with the common good, it reveals a lack of self-awareness and complex self-perceptions. These are key elements that distort one's sense of meaning and purpose in life. Today, people frequently justify irrational moral beliefs and ideals. We tend to engage more in self-deception, self-incoherence, and denial of existential truths. The moral sickness in society is worsening because of these self-deceptions and the refusal to accept the existential truth.

The moral sickness in society is most clearly seen through the harmful effects of social disintegration in modern society. We often fail to realize that this social breakdown stems from individuals' experiences of self-disintegration. With a unified sense of self in social values and attitudes, there is a decline in empathy, mutual understanding, and reciprocity in modern society, which accelerates and sustains social disintegration. Despite living in a world where cultures blend and barriers are broken down, the human dignity of those who are different is often violated. In daily life, people usually position themselves as intolerant of differences and are increasingly unwilling to respect diversity and equality. The moral self limits perspectives that one needs to bridge divides and build social cohesion.

The health research literature indicates that moral illness in the postmodern world underlies nearly all public safety issues and health emergencies in society. Researchers have found that front-line healthcare providers often treat patients whose health problems stem more from moral pain and suffering than from natural causes.[4] A stagnant, weak, rigid, deviant, and harmful moral self contributes to moral disease as a public health crisis more than any social or cultural factor. People's moral pain and suffering impose a significant financial burden on the public health system. However, public health policies rarely prioritize moral health.

The widespread moral pain and suffering experienced by people, despite all scientific and technological advances aimed at improving human life, highlight the need for public policies at local, national, and international levels to play a crucial role in eliminating moral disease. The harm caused by moral disease in our world demonstrates that it is a pressing global health crisis of unprecedented magnitude. Yet, at the same time, governments worldwide ignore this public health crisis as if it were nothing.

Many modern social thinkers and health experts argue that the state of society and the postmodern world can be more characterized by moral disease than moral health. The acute crisis of moral decay in our world can be described as a warning signal for impending catastrophes worldwide. Numerous politicians, civic and religious leaders, and public health officials identify several unique issues in modern times as a public health crisis – such as gun violence – but they overlook the deep moral pain and suffering that underlie these

---

[4] Campbell, SM et.al. A Broader Understanding of Moral Distress. American Journal of Bioethics, Vol 16; 2016

problems.

We are blind to our own moral pain and suffering, and even more so to the consequences it has on society. There is less awareness of how moral disease spreads in society compared to other familiar or emerging infectious diseases. The intense, life-draining, and stifling effects of moral pain and suffering in our times have likely not been experienced by previous generations. Spiritual and moral experts believe this is because we poorly aspire to live guided by principles of high-mindedness, interdependence, human solidarity, and virtues like altruism, tolerance, and compassion. We have lost our orientation toward others in human life.

Some argue that the logical solution to society's problems today lies in restoring traditional morality. However, others contend that the culture of the postmodern world faces highly complex challenges in the moral realm of human life. They argue that conventional morality is becoming ineffective in addressing these issues.

What is conspicuous is that traditional morality no longer effectively prevents the deterioration of the moral environment in society. Moral chaos characterizes the current state of human life in the world, rather than moral health, enhancing the welfare of society and humanity. Each day, we unknowingly follow paths that undermine the integrity of the moral self and weaken moral health. Today, people's values, goals, and lifestyles often lead to moral pain, suffering, and illnesses, rather than fostering robustness of moral well-being, which could also support their mental well-being. The need for moral resilience to develop mental resilience and holistic health is the pressing issue of the hour. The state of moral health or disease has a direct impact on individual well-being and society.

The primary strategy to combat the crisis of moral disease in both individuals and society is to emphasize the importance of cultivating higher-order personhood. Evidence from everyday life suggests that moral health is often neglected without intentional self-development. We fail to incorporate moral purposes into our daily thoughts, feelings, and actions due to inadequate self-awareness. Mental health experts maintain that many people do not sufficiently address moral issues and dilemmas that can harm them through indifference. Humanists observe that individuals often lack the willingness to assess their moral selves regularly. Health professionals believe our moral health development does not sufficiently drive us in daily healthcare. Social reformers find that few people strive for higher ideals and goals in life.

Additionally, we tend to be content with a static human consciousness through which we operate in everyday life. It generates the rigid moral self that is focused on a black-and-white world of good and evil or right and wrong, but not higher-order personhood. Without evolving in human consciousness, we do not mature in the moral self. Essentially, without a higher-order personhood, we do not cultivate the higher cognitive and emotional skills that characterize a mature moral self.

Every day, people struggle to recognize the value and importance of moral health and to commit to it. The malign influences of modern human culture and the denial of objective existential truth hinder people from engaging in self-evaluation and self-regulation. They have a limited understanding and knowledge of their own moral identity and moral self as a person. Without valuing and appreciating moral health, there will inevitably be processes of disintegration within one's personhood and a chaotic sense of self, which essentially indicates that the stage is set for a degenerate moral environment in society.

MORAL CONSCIENCE VS MORAL CONSCIOUSNESS

The moral conscience is deeply ingrained in the average person's mind, guiding their everyday thoughts, feelings, values, attitudes, and behaviors. It is formed through internalization and habituation of societal morals during our upbringing. The moral conscience influences how we are conditioned to think, choose, and decide what constitutes moral behavior. It functions as an internal judge, allowing us to evaluate ourselves. People rely on their moral conscience as a standard to hold themselves accountable for their actions, but it can be made rigid or flexible to suit their needs. Moral conscience can modify people's values, beliefs, perceptions, choices, and decisions to align with their desired behaviors, even if those actions conflict with moral principles or ideals of conscience.

For nearly everyone, moral conscience functions as the only resource for daily moral reasoning and is considered the only tool for evaluating a moral self. It is believed to help us develop moral health. However, our personal life stories often reveal that moral conscience is a weak resource for this development. We lie, cheat, steal, covet, abuse, and indulge in many habits, tendencies, and behaviors that are deeply harmful to moral health. Furthermore, historical evidence shows that moral conscience has been claimed by some of the most reprehensible and morally repugnant people in history: tyrants, dictators, murderers, bigots, racists, and others. For example, Otto Eichmann, the Nazi officer, testified that his conscience was the moral compass for his actions. People's moral conscience has been used to justify the slave trade, the Crusades, ethnic cleansing, genocide, and wars.

In daily life, conventional morality serves as the main moral framework through which almost everyone develops their moral self. It encompasses a range of ideas, from religious to legal, social, harmful, and noble. Conventional morality primarily guides an individual's moral self and holds them responsible for their actions through moral conscience. It establishes the standards for what is considered acceptable behavior for someone to be seen as a moral person in society. The moral standards of a person's conscience are mainly determined and enforced by religion and law.

Humans are a unique species in many ways. We are the only species with religion. We are the only ones who find the origins of moral order in the supernatural. Religion provides frameworks of beliefs and behaviors, labeling some as good, bad, and evil, as well as distinguishing between truths and untruths, right and wrong, and sacred and profane. This illustrates how moral conscience operates in everyday life. Moral conscience is fundamentally a construct of religion used to distinguish moral polarities, helping individuals judge and condemn themselves and others.

More than any other social institution, religion plays a crucial role in shaping moral conscience, and its beliefs form the foundation of conventional morality. It establishes moral standards and guides the behaviors of a moral self. However, religion elevates its moral ideals, values, and motivations within a closed system, leaving no room for genuine dissent. The moral absolutism of religion halts critical thinking and fosters moral rationality based on absolutes. These create division in the moral sphere between "they" and "us" by blaming, judging, and condemning. Nonetheless, it must be acknowledged that any form of moral absolutism—whether cultural, legal, or religious—fails to recognize that critical thinking, intuition, and deeper insight are relevant to the moral self and can improve moral well-being.

We know that non-moral and immoral people have misused religion. Many historical and current events demonstrate that the moral self people develop through religion often leads to social intolerance, violence, communal tensions, and hostilities. It has also justified the persecution and eradication of religious heretics and the destruction of ethnic minorities. Many wars and acts of mass killing by suicide bombers originate from religious absolutism.

Nevertheless, even the most repressive religious cultures produced non-conforming thinkers who challenged and opposed conventional morality through their actions. They morally positioned themselves to refute and dispute the absolutism of moral ideals. They demonstrated the ability to recognize and value common humanity over the habituation of moral conscience generated by conventional morality.

Voices opposing moral conscience reflect a natural development of moral consciousness that can never be silenced. Such individuals demonstrate that the epistemic function of conscience does not necessarily align with the epistemic role of moral consciousness, which is a result of higher human intellectual faculties that shape behaviors to define true humanity. The functional role of human intellect, including reason, intuition, and perception, is vital to our daily human experience.

Yet another institution that powerfully shapes moral conscience is the common law. Few people realize that traditional morality is embedded in the legal system. Through laws, society reflects moral ideals and standards of conventional morality that influence people's behavior. From a legal perspective, individuals accept the moral standards established by the legal system, which allows actions to be judged as right or wrong, good or evil, praiseworthy or blameworthy. The legal system enforces moral conscience through external coercion and the fear of punishment.

Furthermore, in the legal system, moral judgments about behavior rely on the concepts of *mens rea* and *actus reus*. Determining moral wrongness and blameworthiness involves analyzing both the outcome of an action and the person's intent according to moral standards and ideals. There is potential for certain loopholes to allow moral conscience to distort moral reasoning and enable individuals to evade moral responsibility, obligation, and duty. We know from daily life experiences that society's laws often fall short in fostering high-level personhood, holistic health, and enhancing the moral environment in society.

The development of the moral self and moral sense by the legal system relies solely on the external motivational force behind behaviors. It is this motivational force that typically fulfills the minimal moral obligation and responsibility. This often results from a blurred moral sense or an avoided moral self, which are created by illogical legal worldviews.

Most legal norms do not influence the more developed moral self and moral abilities; instead, these undermine the nurturance of moral health. Furthermore, the legal system is filled with laws that are socially irrelevant and have little impact on the moral reasoning behind people's behaviors. Critics of our modern legal system argue that it is ill-suited for scientific rationalism and the diversity of moral frameworks of heterogeneous societies in our contemporary world. They claim it causes more harm than good to individuals, communities, and humanity.

The moral prohibitions, inhibitions, and constraints of traditional morality are easily justified and rationalized. People often fail to recognize the inconsistency between the behaviors they justify and the truths, facts, and reality they encounter. Traditional morality only encourages feelings of approval or disapproval of their own flawed behavior and that of others. Conventional morality is indifferent to the objectivity and rationality of factual truth in guiding thoughts and actions.

It is widely recognized that societal and cultural expectations of a moral conscience are crucial to everyone's human development. It is also widely accepted that guidance from moral conscience is essential to human life. The moral principles, ideals, and values of traditional morality that govern human life are embedded in the collective thinking of humanity. However, what we often overlook is that conventional morality, which is based on social, legal, and religious systems—the foundations of the moral conscience—is filled with outdated ideas, distorted worldviews, irrational beliefs, and false idealism.

This moral conscience is proving to be not only ineffective but also a disruptive influence on individuals across all areas of modern life. It more often suppresses self-evolution, psychosocial maturity, as well as civility and human decency. More importantly, the moral conscience we engage with in life appears to hinder higher-order thinking, innate human moral capacities, and the social sensitivity necessary for our times. To understand and grasp the moral sense and moral motivation that moral consciousness provides, a person's moral conscience requires careful examination.

Ordinary people generally believe that everyone is born with a moral conscience rather than with the potential to evolve in moral consciousness. Few realize that, beyond conscience, it is the influence of moral consciousness that has prompted dutiful objections, driven the search for the whole truth, led public protests, and even put people in deadly danger.

Although we live in a world shaped by scientific and technological progress, the subconscious influence of moral conscience negatively impacts people's rational, logical, and pragmatic thinking in everyday life. These influences shape our relationship patterns. They often cause individuals to judge, blame, condemn, and ignore the present truth, facts, and reality directly in front of them.

We often overlook the fact that our everyday moral conscience reduces the ontological reality of human life and the metaphysical nature of humanity, on which human consciousness and a richer human life rely. People who embrace the metaphysical aspects of human nature are continually evolving in their consciousness, which in turn impacts the quality of their lives. They feel less constrained by the moral ideals, purposes, and pressures of moral conscience.

The evolving human consciousness is essential to explore and understand one's moral conscience. It helps a person uncover subconscious illogical ideas, irrational reasoning, and faulty assumptions that influence daily thinking, values, attitudes, and behaviors. This paves the way for the growth of one's acute awareness of the moral entity when responding in moral matters.

Moral conscience needs to be demystified. It is widely believed that humans innately possess it. While it can negatively impact their moral well-being, people cannot completely detach themselves from their moral conscience. Ordinary individuals often find themselves caught up in irrational feelings of conscience shaped by traditional morality.

Moral conscience is the only human phenomenon in health that tends to evoke reverence rather than questions. It does not undergo deliberate scrutiny from people. Neither the historical development of conscience in an individual nor the societal and cultural factors influencing its development are ever examined.

Moral conscience and moral consciousness form a system of information that guides our understanding of existential experiences and influences decision-making on moral issues. Many view the epistemic role of moral conscience as rigid and limiting, which can lead to a flimsy, uncertain moral self that we carry throughout life. It often causes subtle adverse effects, primarily on emotional and social health, and also impacts physical and mental well-being. Additionally, in today's cultural landscape, moral conscience struggles to contain social, cultural, and political forces that promote harmful behaviors.

In contrast, the epistemic role and function of moral consciousness draw on the powers of higher cognitive abilities, such as reason, intuition, sense perception, and elevated affective capacities, including sensibility and empathetic amiability. It is receptive and open to truth and reality, standing in the face of a person during moral dilemmas. Moral consciousness differs significantly from the former in that it is rooted in the present moment of life and relies on human higher intellectual faculties. It consolidates information that it may either store or reject.

Many scholars and scientists believe there is a clear distinction between moral conscience and moral consciousness. The main difference is that conscience requires only minimal cognitive ability to act, while moral consciousness involves the mind constantly receiving, recognizing, and analyzing moral issues and dilemmas.

Moral conscience forms the moral sense and motivation, shaped by upbringing, society, and culture, to express one's moral self. It depends on past moral knowledge gained through internalization and habituation during a person's development. However, with moral consciousness, the moral sense and motivation emerge from a thorough understanding of the truth.

Moral rules and imperatives limit the thoughts within the moral conscience. As a result, a person can easily become disconnected from a fuller understanding of what truly constitutes truth and reality in the present moment. Moral consciousness interacts with current existential truth and reality, shaping moral sense and motivation for behavior.

Moral consciousness is notably adaptable, holistic, and objectively rational. Daily experiences often show that moral conscience can push us to the edge of subjectivity and disbelief. Similarly, some might argue that moral consciousness also causes individuals to operate on a narrow edge of subjectivity. However, the very nature of human consciousness is to go beyond mental limits in understanding and perceiving truth and reality. In daily life, conventional morality may often seem to lose its meaning, purpose, and objectivity in our moral sense. However, moral consciousness is driven by the "truth" phenomenon, which infuses moral sense and motivation and is essential for a relevant moral response.

Typically, people rely on moral ideals and rules of conventional morality when they prioritize moral conscience. They use a moral conscience that only guides behaviors and interactions within the framework of moral imperatives. These individuals base their moral self on abstract moral ideals and principles, many of which are irrelevant in the moral context of our world. In contrast, moral consciousness involves the present-moment existential moral truth and reality, which are essential for objectivity in the moral sphere. It is driven by selflessness, empathetic amiability, and humaneness that support meaning-making in more complex human experiences.

In this context, moral consciousness is viewed as the first level, with moral conscience as the second, in the development of moral health. The reward and punishment system in traditional morality can only offer limited help in actively promoting moral health. We all need moral consciousness to shape the moral self that reflects higher personhood and encourages better behavior based on the principles of interdependence and human solidarity. Personal integrity and character, therefore, can never be just about pursuing one's moral status in society but are about growing into a holistic selfhood rooted in higher-order personhood.

The easiest way to show how the two differ is that conventional morality issued from conscience, which allowed slave-owning as a natural form of possession; however, helping slaves escape or ending the inhumane practice required moral consciousness. Or moral conscience makes us condemn a hungry man stealing a loaf of bread, but moral consciousness leads us to consider the unjust economic system causing the problem.

There is much about human life that we are relatively unaware of. In matters of moral health, we walk a fine line between subjectivity and personal tendencies when relying on the standards of moral conscience. To objectify one's moral self with a set of standards, rules, and regulations from conventional morality is to dismiss the moral content of human consciousness.

Moral consciousness helps examine moral dilemmas that are often limited by the scope of moral conscience. It influences a person's moral motivation and behavior differently from moral conscience. Moral

23

consciousness is about how moral strength develops through people's immediate experiences of being in the world.

Since ancient times, it has been widely believed that humans possess an innate moral nature and that moral content is inherently embedded in human consciousness. Aristotle stated: "We have the virtues (which I refer to as moral consciousness) neither by nor contrary to our nature. Our nature is designed to receive them." Modern science supports this by showing that moral consciousness has a neural basis, indicating that human consciousness is rooted in neurobiology. Whether directly or indirectly, the concept of the "moral" is always present in human consciousness. Our ideals, thoughts, and dreams across various domains—material, social, economic, political, ecological—are all integrated within consciousness.

Experts believe that the "moral content" in human consciousness comes from either moral conscience or moral consciousness. They also highlight that the "moral content" of human consciousness includes both what is learned through conventional morality and the self-evident "moral truth" that is intuitively perceived and deeply felt. The "moral content" of a person's moral consciousness is different from moral conscience because it can create the potential for moral sense and moral motivation that go beyond what personal moral conscience establishes. The moral content of consciousness filters out unimportant or irrelevant aspects of moral sense, including moral ideals of conventional morality, and instead focuses on moral issues and challenges.

Moral consciousness involves the brain mechanisms of complex cognitive and emotional functions that resist reducing moral sense to fixed ideals, principles, or simple rules and regulations. Modern sciences reveal that the intellectual complexities of knowledge, reason, and judgment involve higher faculties, such as intuition, sense perception, and deeper insight. These intellectual faculties enhance the "moral content" in a person's evolving consciousness and are not rigidly fixed, as occurs with moral conscience. The cognitive function of moral consciousness is essential for logical thinking, decision-making, and responsible actions in the moral realm. A higher tendency for self-regulation and self-control is influenced more by one's moral consciousness than by moral conscience.

In literature, moral sense is described as the instinctual ability to perceive and avoid harm. The origin of moral sense can stem from internal, external, or both internal and external sources. Typically, people's moral sense and motivation are influenced by their moral conscience. However, a well-developed moral sense stems from higher cognitive skills, such as intuition, rather than just moral rules. Some experts believe that humans have an innate moral sense encoded in DNA.

We will now examine the brain's higher cognitive functions to better understand how moral conscience and moral consciousness function as information systems in the decision-making process for daily actions that affect moral health.

The highest level of brain function is cognition—the thinking process.[5] The experience of consciousness involves the cognitive function of attention, which gathers information, and alertness, to focus and select specific information while ignoring others. Consciousness is responsible for attention and alertness, both of which are necessary for the awareness skill. The brain has the ability for self-awareness, meaning the awareness of one's cognitive and mental processes. Self-awareness is a higher form of consciousness that supports the development of self-identity.

At a higher level of cognitive function, consciousness encompasses the introspective awareness of oneself, characterized by self-awareness. This contemplative quality is essential to moral consciousness. While moral conscience relates to a person's psychological state, moral consciousness is associated with neurobiology. From a clinical neurologic perspective, attention

---

[5] Benson, F. The Neurology of Thinking. Oxford Press (1994)
Buss AH. Personality: Evolutionary Heritage and Human Distinctiveness, Lawrence Erlbaum Associates (1988)

and alertness are the first prerequisites for developing moral health. It is a product of human consciousness.

Neuroscience has uncovered a neural basis for consciousness. The evidence indicates that consciousness happens when information becomes widely accessible to multiple brain systems—an event generated by a network of neurons, mainly in the prefrontal cortex, which broadcasts signals across different brain areas.[6] Researchers have demonstrated that consciousness is an active mental process involving various anatomical and chemical components within the brain. Neuroscience explains that both conscious and unconscious states depend on complex interactions within a network of brain regions known as the ascending reticular activating system (ARAS).

Neuroscience highlights that cognition – the thinking process behind our self-awareness – involves several parallel brain activities. When we focus on self-awareness and awareness of daily actions, our consciousness encompasses multiple aspects, including sensation, perception—which is the abstraction of sensation—memory, and motivation. Self-awareness emphasizes moral concerns and the implications of life experiences through moral consciousness. However, we often find self-awareness to be elusive. Scientists have demonstrated that impaired attention, inefficient memory, loss of inhibitory control, and difficulty detecting novelty can disrupt sustained cognitive function. In daily life, this results in impaired self-awareness, leading to a reduced ability for conscious self-evaluation and appropriate behavioral adjustments.

The moral implications of life experiences are rooted in those experiences themselves. When one's moral sense develops from the continuous flow of human consciousness, which is always present, it influences the moral self in different ways. Moral consciousness allows us to see clearly who we are and who we can become. Self-awareness is crucial to our self-identity, which

---

[6] Dehaene, S. et.al. A neuronal model of a global workspace in effortful cognitive tasks. PNAS (Vol 95), November 1998

constantly evolves as part of the ongoing story of our lives. When we know who we are, feel comfortable with that, and act with self-awareness, moral consciousness often takes priority over moral conscience in our choices, decisions, and actions. Moral consciousness can help develop a moral self that is different from the one shaped only by traditional morality. The latter moral self is more common, while the former tends to be less evident in society.

We must see it as our duty to uncover the ideas within our moral conscience to understand the moral self that is part of our identity. We need to identify the moral sense and motivation behind our daily choices and decisions to develop the potential of the moral self through moral consciousness, especially when addressing the problems and challenges of the postmodern world. A more developed moral self results from the perfect integration and integrity of rationality and emotions. It is guided by the universal "code of rules and prohibitions" embedded in human DNA, which determines what is right and wrong based on the moral content of human consciousness.

People's moral self and moral sense always develop and grow through moral consciousness. They are neither fixed nor unchanging, unlike when governed solely by moral conscience. This moral self and moral sense can be altered, modified, and adjusted to align with one's moral purpose in life and to conform to higher ideals, values, and beliefs. Although capable of integrating rules based on conventional morality's system of reward and punishment, moral consciousness is not limited by the standards and ideals of traditional morality, as it reflects the intentions of moral conscience.

Moral conscience is an insufficient resource for self-regulation and self-control of everyday behaviors. When driven by a visceral chain of more tempting hedonic motivations, moral conscience remains ineffective despite its set of moral ideals guiding a person's moral sense and motivation. In contrast, moral consciousness encourages the tendency to resist acting on impulses that lead to harmful behaviors. It enables people to consistently experience psychological discomfort from thoughts that precede actions, negatively impacting their moral health.

The global hedonic culture, which blurs the line between right and wrong, good and evil, is effectively weakening the moral sense that guides behaviors for personal and collective well-being. Additionally, people often experience mental fatigue from moral ideals that feel more like a punitive system, causing guilt, shame, and self-abhorrence. In a world where moral sense is ambiguous and the concept of a moral self is distorted, our ability to self-regulate and control behavior relies more on moral consciousness than on moral conscience.

Everyone experiences an ongoing incarnation in the world. People who focus on self-awareness have an open-ended life story, where the "self" is the main protagonist. When someone is supported by self-awareness, there are evolving cognitive and emotional processes that help the person evaluate and develop their moral self. This causes the individual to change their self-identity in the narrative to include a constantly evolving moral self. As humans, we have higher intellectual abilities that enable us to distinguish truth from falsehood and fact from fiction, pushing the limits of our moral capacities and forming a moral self that drives us to act and behave differently.

The fundamental nature of human consciousness is to inquire, to want to know, and to find meaning. Truth is the one thing through which everything in life is connected, has meaning, and is destined for. Human consciousness alone keeps the truth alive and active in us. The "truth" phenomenon is the driving force behind the human need to establish cause-and-effect connections behind everything. As a form of self-awareness, consciousness is the ontological basis for human life. Human consciousness is the potential we always have to know the objective truth. Essentially, human consciousness involves the "truth" phenomenon in the current life experience. To cultivate moral health, one must depend on the "truth" phenomenon.

The "truth" phenomenon reflects the idea that when people develop moral health, their moral sense emerges from higher cognitive and emotional abilities. Truth influences an individual's moral sense differently than standards, ideals, and rules. The "truth" phenomenon is filtered through the interaction of internal and external environments via reason, insight, intuition, instinct, and sense perception. Unlike ideals, principles, rules, and standards of moral conscience, the "truth" phenomenon helps shape moral sense.

Innate abilities, such as intuition, instinct, insight, and sensory perception, fuel moral consciousness. It serves as the channel of moral human nature that differentiates humans from animals through their unique moral capacities. Moral consciousness requires an individual's moral sense to heighten their awareness of the truth in each present moment.

In our times, the "truth" phenomenon has become even more essential to moral understanding because it helps us recognize the importance of confronting serious dangers lurking beneath moral issues in our world, which is leading humanity into moral chaos. Moral consciousness, influenced by inherent higher cognitive abilities, develops the "truth" phenomenon in every present moment. In contrast, moral conscience, which has developed as a tool within the family, community, and society, may or may not include the "truth" phenomenon.

So, essentially, the moral self and moral sense of a person are not only developed capacities, socially anchored and constructed, but also are always flexible with the phenomenon of "truth" in moral consciousness. Additionally, moral consciousness drives a person toward a deeper understanding of the truth of moral issues that influence one's moral self and affect the behaviors impacting others.

However, we also know that the "truth" phenomenon tends to stay elusive. Usually, truth is a slippery phenomenon we find hard to grasp and understand. We can only approximate the truth. For example, when someone closes their eyes with the palms of their hands, it is dark. This makes sense because no light is entering, but it isn't the whole truth. Infrared light exists; it has a slightly longer wavelength than visible light. Warm objects, including the human body, constantly emit infrared light. However, human eyes are not as sensitive to infrared light as they are to visible light. If they were, we would be blinded even with our eyelids closed, just from the light emitted by our own eyes.

The "truth" phenomenon arises from conflicting forces within a person's mind, often compared to the light at the end of a tunnel. Its elusive and approximate nature frequently causes people to hesitate to confront, pursue, understand, or measure it. Consciousness helps us grasp the phenomenon of "truth" with its nuances, unlike conscience. However, consciousness isn't just nonsense about truth. It encourages a deep understanding and assessment of current human experiences, consistently revealing the "truth" phenomena of that particular moment, which are otherwise difficult to perceive when we depend solely on conscience.

We must recognize that moral consciousness alone allows us to interpret the "truth" phenomena, helping to develop our moral self and guiding our moral sense in choices, decisions, and actions. Essentially, moral consciousness is a form of self-awareness in which future actions are based on truth, reflecting how one perceives oneself as a human being in the world. It is fundamental to self-identity, personality style, character traits, and a well-integrated, holistic life. Therefore, making pragmatic and realistic observations in daily life is a responsibility to the truth of the present moment, leading to a richer human experience. Moral health involves continually confronting the truth as it unfolds to understand the "as-is" human existence. It develops as observations lead to clearer perception, reason, and intuition, enabling better judgment and appropriate actions in the moment.

Moral consciousness is an endless source of energy to improve ourselves and humanity. One of the highest forms of human consciousness occurs when we can enhance our ability to honor our humanity and feel empowered to overcome self-centered thinking, thereby fostering empathetic amiability and human solidarity. While moral conscience offers guidance on how people should behave morally based on ideals and principles, it is moral consciousness that enables us to systematically evaluate the moral issues we face on a daily basis. Consciousness is fundamental to the powers of moral human nature. In moments of moral consciousness, we are challenged to look inward—at the inner self and core realities—and discover the dignity and worthiness of being human. Only then can we extend this dignity and worthiness to others.

Evolving human consciousness offers a path to realize this ideal within ourselves and throughout humanity. While people are driven by a desire to do what is right and good, they often fall short due to a lack of self-regulation and self-control. Therefore, each person has a responsibility to uncover and develop the moral consciousness of both who we are and who we aim to become.

Whether intentionally or not, we all evaluate our moral selves in everyday life. It guides us toward what is considered a "good," "virtuous," "just," "right," or "ethical" way to act. This moral self-assessment encourages behaviors that promote empathy, fairness, and altruism toward others. Moral self-evaluation is a key trait of healthy individuals who are capable and willing to acknowledge their responsibility for their choices, decisions, and actions.

The moral self-evaluation we perform can be guided either by external standards of normative morality or by personal ideals, aspirations, values, and beliefs. Usually, everyday moral self-assessments influence one's motivation, choices, and decisions for actions and behaviors based on moral ideals of conscience that were formed a long time ago. However, moral consciousness conducts moral self-evaluation independently of the social context, specific norms, or the identities that we have developed through moral conscience. It is rooted in current moral entities and realities.

A complete moral self-evaluation, undertaken with moral consciousness, reveals subconscious illogical ideas, reasoning, and assumptions that directly or indirectly influence everyday thinking, values, attitudes, and behaviors. The process involves deeper cognition through sense perception, intuition, and insight. It includes examining the psyche's content related to one's inner core realities that impact the moral self and moral sense. This helps strengthen the ability to stay firm in one's present-focused moral sense and moral self when acting.

Moral consciousness is always shaped by a person's inner-core realities and current life experiences. It is an existential phenomenon that develops through everyday living. Unlike moral conscience, which stems from fixed ideals, moral indoctrination, prescriptions, and regulations, moral consciousness is more adaptable. Therefore, moral self-evaluation is influenced differently by moral conscience and moral consciousness because each perceives one's inner-core realities in its own way.

When a person's moral self is formed by moral conscience, it is judged by external standards rather than by internal core realities. When guided by individual moral awareness, it can help reveal the true self, confront the pseudo-self, and analyze the uncertain ideas of moral conscience concerning core inner realities.

Every person can cultivate moral consciousness, enabling us to broaden our moral comprehension through life experiences. It is not acquired via education, laws, or social and cultural teachings. Instead, moral consciousness evolves through ordinary daily life experiences, bolstered by higher mental abilities such as awareness, perception, insight, and intuition. It involves an ever-evolving human consciousness, triggering self-evolution and psychosocial maturity.

Human life is built on the framework of interpersonal relationships. Both positive and negative interactions shape the fabric of our lives. Moral consciousness enhances our understanding of human connections. It motivates us to be other-oriented and act in ways that serve the common good and uphold human dignity in ourselves and others. Emile Durkheim introduced the term 'sociology of morality,' which, according to today's health experts, relates to the state of society's moral consciousness.[7] The survival and growth of any society depend more on its ability to recognize and regulate human life through the moral content of people's consciousness than on traditional morality. It is through everyday interactions that people foster moral health by strengthening the sense of a common humanity through amiable interpersonal bonds.

Moral consciousness is both collective and individual. It conducts a thorough moral evaluation of personal, social, and cultural factors. It acknowledges the moral sense that guides our actions toward others in what is proper and essential. Today, we should judge human progress not by more achievements but by fewer societal problems and global issues. Based on our observations of people's moral selves, the mental process of moral conscience is as complex as human diversity. Unexamined moral assumptions rooted in traditional morality, particularly regarding issues of diversity in our world, require critical analysis through the lens of moral consciousness.

Today, we live amidst diverse cultures with varying moral views and worldviews. We must respect everyone's welfare and dignity, but conventional moral values can't be universally applied to all people, cultures, or situations. Developing moral consciousness is crucial for cultivating a social attitude that aligns with meaningful moral objectives. This awareness enables individuals to recognize human interconnectedness and collective responsibility as vital moral principles. Shared responsibility plays a crucial role in inspiring moral actions that promote well-being on personal and societal levels. In daily life, the moral sense, rooted in moral consciousness, differs from moral conscience primarily in its emphasis on interconnectedness and solidarity through empathy, compassion, tolerance, love, and mutual support.

Today's human culture is a melting pot of social diversity, which brings varying attitudes and views on what constitutes good, bad, correct, or wrong behavior. As a result, moral conscience can sometimes be ineffective or

---

[7] Durkheim, E. Emile Durkheim on Morality and Society (Heritage of Sociology Series). University of Chicago Press, 1973

unsuitable for interdependence and human solidarity, the essential life principles in the postmodern times. Its ideals often fail to achieve the intended outcomes of a healthier humanity and a better world order. Conversely, moral consciousness taps into our deeper insights, intuitions, and practical wisdom, enabling us to comprehend moral truths and act upon them. It operates dynamically, flowing from external influences to internal understanding and back, constantly renewing our moral awareness to confront urgent moral dilemmas and resolve pressing issues. Hence, moral consciousness provides a more precise approach to examining questions of good and evil, right and wrong by understanding and learning from the present moment's existential truths, realities, and human complexities. To develop moral health, we must broaden and deepen our fact-based understanding of moral issues through ongoing dialogue with our real-time lived experiences.

Growing moral health depends on a commitment to moral well-being at personal, societal, and global levels. Some social scientists suggest that a healthy person should be characterized more by the ability to respect the welfare, dignity, and self-worth of everyone, as well as the self-regulatory ability to avoid harming and humiliating others. Developing moral consciousness must be a collective effort of society. We need to build the moral capacities to consciously enhance the quality of human life in our world, which in turn strengthens the moral well-being of humanity. Experts believe that as society progresses in developing moral consciousness, it will overcome moral chaos and the degraded moral climate worldwide. People's moral consciousness will guide their self-evaluation to aim for the humane in all circumstances. Their moral self-actualization will not be limited by cultural values or traditional morality but will reflect higher-order personhood, revealing psychosocial maturity at all times.

THE MORAL HUMAN NATURE

What makes humans distinctly moral beings has long fascinated and challenged scholars in the fields of religion, philosophy, and psychology. Scientists, researchers, scholars, and everyday people continue to work to understand the origins of moral human nature, both at the level of universal foundations and cultural variations.

Since the dawn of human civilization, it has been believed that humans are inherently moral. The moral phenomenon has always been seen as defining what it means to be human. It has consistently been argued that human moral nature elevates humans within the animal kingdom. From ancient times, human moral abilities and tendencies have been metaphorically regarded as the earthly signature of the human soul.

It is natural for humans to seek moral living. We evaluate human life based on moral standards. What makes us valuable as humans is actions guided by moral judgment and purpose. It is hard to picture any individual or society without some form of moral reasoning. Social scientists inform us that, despite cultural and personal differences, everyone functions within a moral framework.

The moral human nature is closely connected to how we understand the meaning and purpose of human life. It is deeply embedded in human experience and always involved in thought, feeling, and behavior. Throughout history, the ideal human life has consistently included the moral self. The moral self is crucial for forming an orientation toward others.

Since the beginning of human civilization, the moral self has been understood as what it takes for a person to be truly human. The moral self defines what it means to be human and how a person lives a human life. It has always been the ideal to live a human life, even at a personal cost, and more so, even at the expense of one's own life. The more people sacrifice self-interest and personal security for the common good, the more they embody the true nature of moral humanity.

The moral self is an essential part of human personhood. It is the core of one's sense of self. The essence of a person's personhood and selfhood is reflected in the moral self. The moral self supports the full functioning of a person's identity and self-awareness. It influences all aspects of life, including lifestyles, self-fulfillment, life goals, aspirations, relationships, and even struggles and problems. The moral self directs human thoughts, feelings, and actions, distinguishing between what is moral and immoral.

How do we tell good from evil, right from wrong, just from unjust, and vice from virtue? An obvious answer is that we have gained the ability through our upbringing. We distinguish between what is acceptable and unacceptable in society by developing a conscience. Moral principles, ideals, values, and rules shape the moral conscience. Throughout human history, various moral ideals, values, and rules for human behavior have been developed to coexist. They become the prerequisites for fitting into society.

In the animal kingdom, only humans prioritize moral and ethical behaviors. Human society expects and enforces standards of morality and ethics. Legal principles and laws are based on society's ethical and moral framework. Conventional morality helps us determine who is acting morally and ethically. Through socialization, we learn to fit into society by adjusting our behaviors and attitudes. Socialization helps us develop a conventional moral framework that guides us to act with a moral self.

However, what we are discovering today is that the moral capacity of human nature cannot be confined to traditional morality. Biological anthropologists explain that the natural evolution of the human species has led to the development of the "moral brain," something not present in other animals. The "moral brain" distinguishes humans from any other creature. The prevailing view in the scientific community is that humans are uniquely endowed with moral abilities in the animal kingdom. Nature has endowed humans with moral capacities to uphold human stature and dignity among animals.

The study of the origins of human moral nature is both ancient and modern. It has been a subject of philosophical inquiry for thousands of years. For example, in ancient India, the Vedic literature highlighted the key difference between humans and animals in terms of the unique human intellectual ability to discriminate and select behaviors. In ancient China, Confucianism emphasized the importance of both nature and nurture in developing moral behaviors. In ancient Greece, in the fictional dialogue of Plato's Meno, the author famously asks Socrates, "Whether virtue is acquired by teaching or by practice; or if neither by teaching nor practice, then whether it comes to man by nature, or in what other way?"

Today, the study of moral human nature is a truly interdisciplinary effort that draws significant contributions from evolutionary biologists, neuroscientists, psychologists, philosophers, legal scholars, and many others. What modern science is starting to reveal is that moral human nature is deeply embedded in the fabric of human nature. Advances in science have given us many reasons to believe that we are getting closer to uncovering the neural substrates that make us moral beings.

In our time, evolutionary scientists reveal that the human moral capacity gradually developed. They provide evidence that the evolution of the human brain led to higher cognitive and emotional abilities, laying the groundwork for moral thinking, emotion, and behavior. Modern science emphasizes that the human brain's networks and mechanisms make humans unique from the rest of the animal kingdom. Additionally, in recent decades, neuroscience has been uncovering the neural networks underlying human moral capacity, which are collectively referred to as the "moral brain."

Today, experts confidently state that the human species has the innate potential to develop abilities to suppress what is less than human. Many argue that the animalistic side in humans is kept in check by innate moral qualities. There is a greater focus on developing innate human moral capacities rather than adhering to prescribed morality. In the postmodern world, scholars and scientists recognize that inherent human moral abilities are better at capturing the essence of humanity—degraded by modern technology—than conventional morality.

The two main lines of scientific inquiry into human moral nature are evolutionary science and neuroscience. Evolutionary biologists help us understand the origin of the brain networks involved in being moral. At the same time, neuroscientists provide evidence of how these brain networks function, especially those unique to humans that shape moral thinking, emotion, and behavior.

Evolutionary Science

Charles Darwin's research found that the key difference between humans and lower animals is a moral sense. Today, his theory of evolution is prompting a reconsideration of the origins of human morality. It has led experts to question the origin of the moral sense, specifically whether it is shaped by biological evolution. How did it develop? When did it appear in human evolution?

There is a growing interest among evolutionary scientists in Darwin's view that the human moral sense is biologically determined. They argue that moral sense, moral motivation, and moral behavior in humans are not solely products of human cultural development, but also stem from biological evolution. Modern-day evolutionary biologists contend that the moral aspect of human nature is rooted in neurobiological makeup.[8]

From the study of human evolution, we are beginning to understand that the ability for moral reasoning in humans is a result of natural selection. Evolutionary biologists believe that moral thinking, feelings, and motivations – the moral brain – have been essential for the survival of the human species. Evolutionary anthropologists argue that the development of the human brain for other-oriented thinking and feeling played a significant role in the evolution of human moral nature.

The experts believe that among our primitive ancestors, certain specific behaviors contributed to their ability to live together successfully. For example, sharing food with those too young or weak to hunt, helping others, sacrificing oneself for the common good, or remaining loyal to one's mate. They assert that the moral aspect of human nature has developed through natural selection and has played a role in the development of the human brain's unique neural network, now called the "moral brain."

What evolutionary scientists are convinced of is that it was a matter of survival that the "moral brain" had to develop. They argue that to survive unpredictable environments, the human brain evolved and created unique neural circuits not found in the rest of the animal kingdom. Evolutionary biologists emphasize that as standards of behavior for communal life improved over time, so did the brain networks in humans evolve, and they continue to develop throughout human history.

Evolutionary anthropologists argue that, through natural selection, the cognitive and emotional abilities of the human brain in our primitive ancestors evolved to higher levels. Although much of the brain's circuits and mechanisms were already inherited from prehuman ancestors, the adaptive learning of these ancestors prewired the human brain to develop the "moral brain" by enhancing cognitive, executive, and motivational capacities.

---

[8] Ayala, FJ. The difference of being human: Morality. PNAS Biological Sciences, (vol 107), May 2010

Scientists believe that the unique "moral brain" in humans results from the natural evolutionary process. Through natural selection, human nature has shaped the "moral brain" within us. Some scientists argue that moral behavior is embedded in human DNA.

The work of evolutionary biologists highlights that, through natural selection, the human brain is wired for moral behaviors. Findings in neuroscience demonstrate that moral reasoning and behavior are biological traits of human nature. The key point is that humans possess neural abilities with biological foundations that have been favored by natural selection. This highlights the crucial role nature plays in shaping human moral capacities and promoting moral well-being.

Neuroscience

Today, neuroscience shows that the "moral brain" serves as the foundation for the moral sense and moral behavior unique to humans. We are beginning to understand with certainty that the "moral brain" in humans involves more advanced cognitive and emotional abilities that evolved through natural selection. There are neural foundations for moral sense and moral actions.

Neuroscience clearly demonstrates that humans possess a moral nature, with a focus on the higher cognitive and emotional functions of the human brain. It is known that in mammals, brain size generally correlates with body size. Relative to body mass, humans have the largest brain. The human brain is not only bigger but also much more complex. The cerebral cortex, where higher cognitive functions are processed, is proportionally much larger in humans than in our primate ancestors.

Neuroscientists emphasize that the most fundamental evolutionary development of the human brain is the advanced intellectual abilities. The mechanisms and functions of the human brain allow us to reason, think abstractly, and imagine realities that are not immediately present. This enables humans to possess a wide range of unique intellectual skills. These skills enable us to create scientific knowledge, forms of art, and literature, as well as to develop social organization and culture.

Modern sciences highlight that the most distinctive functional features of the human mind are self-awareness and awareness of one's own mortality, the reality of one's death. This is a uniquely human ability intrinsic to human nature. Cultural anthropologists emphasize that this has led to the development of morality, ethics, and religion in human life. Human intellectual faculties are crucial for forming moral capacity and are fundamental to developing a moral self. The moral self of a person is an integral part of human nature through innate moral ability.

The moral capacities inherent in human nature help distinguish humans from animals. Morality has long been seen as a feature that separates humanity from the rest of the animal kingdom. However, it is common to find authors who attribute moral selfhood to animals. They argue that some animals possess moral emotions like sympathy, empathy, and patience, and are willing to help other animals. They provide prima facie evidence to support this claim.

Though some people may project the "moral nature" onto other animals, we know that, unlike humans, animals cannot explicitly reason about right and wrong, good and bad, just and unjust, vice and virtue. What makes humans the only moral beings is their capacity for abstract higher-order thinking.

There is neuroscientific evidence that moral emotion, moral reasoning, and moral motivation in moral behaviors have neural foundations. Neuroscientists have identified a brain network that influences a person's moral well-being. Neuroscience shows that the "moral brain" involves higher cognitive and emotional processes of the human mind. Human moral nature relies on this brain network to guide moral behavior.

All animals display certain typical behaviors. For instance, we think of dogs as loyal and sheep as meek. This is because animal behaviors are rooted in nature. Human behaviors are also rooted in human nature. Human behavior is just as much a part of the natural order as the existence of the human species.

Evolutionary psychologists have identified inborn aspects of human behavior. They have found that human infants are born with cognitions and motivations that incline them toward pro-social feelings. Humans are naturally predisposed to moral behavior because of the ability to experience pro-social emotions, such as empathy. Research in human development provides evidence that, from infancy, humans are capable of offering comfort and assistance to others in emotional distress.

Like the rest of the animal kingdom, humans are hardwired for behaviors.[9] However, even though humans are wired for behaviors, these behaviors cannot be viewed uniformly. A person's unique genetic inheritance does not make everyone's behaviors similar. Human behaviors range from vicious cruelty to deep compassion, and understanding this range is essential for assessing moral health.

In recent decades, scientists, researchers, and scholars have emphasized the importance of people's moral consciousness in developing and maintaining a mature moral self. Moral consciousness is vital for cultivating moral health and preventing moral disease within oneself. In literature, experts consider the moral content of human consciousness to be moral consciousness. Neuroscience reveals that human consciousness arises from a complex neurobiological process. The brain mechanisms underlying consciousness are crucial for developing the moral capacities needed to foster moral health.

Neuroscience emphasizes that to develop a moral sense—fostering appropriate behaviors that enhance moral health—there must be increased activity in the action-perception brain mechanism. This involves the brain's higher cognitive functions, including attention, meaning, intention, and goal setting. An individual's level of consciousness influences these functions. Higher levels of human consciousness help us become more aware, attentive,

---

[9] Decety J & Cowell JM, <u>Our Brains are wired for Morality</u>. Frontiers, March 2016

and able to understand the "as-is" truth of the present moment.

The state of moral consciousness reflects higher cognitive abilities such as intuition, insight, and sense perception, which help us understand and interpret everyday experiences to develop a more refined moral self. It enables us to adopt a broader perspective beyond just moral rules. Usually, the moral sense and motivation behind our actions are not instinctive but are shaped through education, law, religion, or social institutions. However, moral consciousness is rooted in human nature and requires ongoing development through self-evolution, triggered by the evolution of human consciousness.

Consciousness is essential to being human. It underpins cognitive functions like awareness, perception, intuition, and similar abilities. Consciousness acts as the pathway for developing the moral capacity of the more advanced moral self. Essentially, this more developed moral self is guided by the universal "code of rules and prohibitions" embedded in human DNA.[10] The more advanced moral self in individuals is rooted in the tendency toward self-awareness, self-evaluation, and self-restraint.

Traditionally, it has been believed that moral behavior depends on a code of values guiding people's choices and actions, and that moral principles and ideals determine the purpose and meaning of human life. However, findings in evolutionary psychology and primatology suggest that emotions, such as kin altruism, reciprocal altruism, and revenge, play a key role in the origins of moral behavior.[11]

There is widespread agreement among researchers that empathy drives prosocial behavior, reduces aggression, and provides the foundation for moral conduct. Empathy is like the brain's "moral sparkplug" in a person. Neuroscience shows that empathy is a brain-related process.

---

[10] Fishe A. Moral Emotions Provide Self-control Needed to Sustain Social Relationships. Self Identity (Vol 1), 2002
[11] Flack, J. & de Wall, FBM. "Any animal whatever": Darwinian building blocks of morality in monkeys and apes. J. Conscious. Stud. (Vol. 7) 2000

From a scientific perspective, Kohlberg's studies marked a significant milestone in the psychological exploration of moral human nature. Kohlberg viewed moral reasoning as a product of cognitive processes that can exist even without any emotion.[12] However, research in evolutionary psychology and primatology indicated that emotions played a crucial role in the origins of moral human nature.[13]

Empathy—the ability to "feel" another's emotional state—is often what leads to moral sense, moral motivation, and moral behavior. It involves the hormone oxytocin, which some scientists refer to as the "moral molecule." Oxytocin is known to increase trust and generosity in some situations and boost envy and bias in others.

From an evolutionary perspective, it is a key molecule found in all mammalian species. It plays a crucial role in mother-offspring bonding and helps reduce fear and anxiety. Evolutionary biologists suggest that empathy initially evolved to enhance parental care in the animal kingdom.

Empathy is essential for prosocial behaviors. Found in many mammals, empathy promotes everyday acts of kindness. While humans empathize with other humans, we also know that many animals do the same. These animals display empathy and engage in prosocial actions. For example, monkeys hug and kiss when others are hurt or scared. Ethologists suggest that this behavior helps alleviate the stress experienced by the victim.

However, among non-human animals, prosocial behaviors are more likely to be shown only toward kin and members of the same social groups. Empathy and prosocial behaviors in humans are not limited to kin and social groups. Empathy gives us the inclination and motivation to help people and cooperate with those who are not related to us at a level that is unmatched in

---

[12] Kohlberg, L. Essays in Moral Development (Vol. 1) The Psychology of Moral Development. Harper & Row, 1984

[13] Trivers, R.L. The evolution of reciprocal altruism. Review of Biology (Vol. 46) 1971, University of Chicago Press Journals

the animal kingdom.

Empathy, recognized in non-human animals, does not require conscious thought or action. The advanced cognitive abilities in humans, along with moral emotions such as empathy, contribute to the development of moral capacities in distinct ways. Humans are distinctly different from all other animals in anatomy, but more importantly, in possessing a unique moral capacity. It is unlike anything in the animal kingdom, thanks to our intellectual abilities. Our metacognitive capacities are what enable us to grow in moral reasoning and moral motivation for everyday behaviors.

The intellectual capacities we possess help us develop intentional behaviors and prevent us from acting solely on animal instincts, which scientists refer to as phylogenetic instincts. Humans are even willing to die for a cause that benefits others, not just themselves. A meaningful human life depends on our intellectual abilities and the enhancement of our moral capacities. As humans, we can only survive and thrive through interactions with others.[14] Almost all everyday actions and thoughts of humans revolve around or respond to others.

The unique moral capacity of human nature influences all aspects of human life. It forms the basis of a moral self in how we act toward others. Through moral reasoning, we recognize that everyday actions have consequences not only for ourselves but also for others. As a highly social species dependent on each other for survival, the human moral capacity is essential to the "good life."

Deepened understanding of morality and moral health

The "moral" is deeply rooted in human nature and integral to the concept of human health. Human nature has an innate capacity to develop moral health. The human intellect provides an inherent ability to cultivate a

---

[14] Tomasello, M & Vaish, A. Origins of human cooperation and morality. Annu. Rev. Psychol. (Vol. 64), 2013.

moral self, playing a crucial role in growing moral health.

All of this originates from the human brain's ability to think abstractly. However, these abstract cognitive skills are built on phylogenetic instincts. A person's instinctual life represents a subjective reality, driven by preprogrammed genetic mechanisms.[15] This accounts for the wide range of behaviors humans can display.

The reason we hold people morally responsible for their behaviors is solely because they have the ability to choose them. The moral capacity to develop a moral self not only sets humans apart from the rest of the animal kingdom but also fundamentally defines what it means to be human. The best use of one's human life depends on how the individual engages with life using their moral capacities.

Being human involves moral duties and responsibilities. That is why, in the animal kingdom, only humans develop lifestyles that adhere to moral standards, ethical guidelines, and legal laws. Moral health and proper healthcare depend on our everyday actions. Human society relies on moral duty, responsibility, and conduct not only to maintain civil and social order but also to advance personal well-being.

The moral capacity also encourages us to be more intentionally interested in and concerned for the well-being of others. The intellectual ability for higher-order thinking helps us act deliberately to override phylogenetic instincts that have negative consequences in human life. There is no better way to connect with one another as humans than through other-oriented behaviors. It relies on us developing our moral capacities and moral self.

It would be misleading to think of moral human nature as solely a result of biological evolution. Although the "moral brain" has evolved through human biological evolution, it has also been shaped and refined by the development of human culture. In fact, we have a "moral brain" that has been

---

[15] Malkemus, S A, Reclaiming Instinct: Exploring the Phylogenetic Unfolding of Animate Being. Journal of Humanistic Psychology (Vol 55.1) 2014

formed over thousands of years through the combination of our genes and cultural influences. It cannot be said that only one or the other has shaped the "moral brain" we carry.

The kind of moral reasoning needed to live together successfully or not depends on the moral self developed through our inherent moral capacities.[16] The moral capacities of our individual brains are fundamentally what enable us to behave the way we do and to care for others as we do. There has been a genetic and cultural evolution that has shaped our unique "moral brain." The functioning of the "moral brain" in people also depends on the cultural environment.

The moral health of a person is shaped by both human nature and human culture. People's moral reasoning and moral self can differ across cultures and evolve over time. For example, bullfighting is viewed as a cruel form of entertainment or even as animal cruelty in some countries, while in others it is not. The example of slavery highlights how moral perceptions have changed over time. Most people today consider it evil, but that was not the case a century ago.

Understanding moral human nature as neurobiologically determined and culturally shaped influences how we consider matters related to building and maintaining moral health. Moral ideals and rules alone cannot be used to evaluate people's moral character. We cannot assess moral health solely based on conventional morality.

Understanding an innate moral nature in humans prompts an examination of moral issues in human life. We will consider several key implications of the moral phenomenon embedded in human nature.

The cognitive functions of the human brain shape an individual's moral capacities and influence moral emotion, moral motivation, and moral behavior, all of which affect moral health. A person's more developed moral capacities

---

[16] Decety, J and Wheatley, T. The Moral Brain: A Multidisciplinary Perspective. Cambridge: MIT Press (2015).

arise from inherent human consciousness.

We all have the inherent moral ability to pursue higher ideals or not. When responding to those who try to harm us, we all possess the innate potential to develop the cognitive and emotional skills necessary for high-minded thinking and a noble spirit manifested by empathetic amiability and altruistic attitudes. The possibility of living a shimmering life exists in everyone if we work toward it.

The moral capacity rooted in prudence, self-control, and advanced self-reflection that enables us to respond appropriately to the present moment is crucial to one's moral self and moral well-being. Neuroscience researchers are helping us better understand the cognitive and emotional processes behind the origins of everyday moral and immoral actions.[17]

Our everyday observations of criminality, corruption, fraud, abuse of power, and similar issues often stop at judging these behaviors as unethical, immoral, or evil. We are quick to condemn such actions and even consider them punishable by law. We tend to assume that everyone knows what is morally "right" rather than morally "wrong" and is free to make their own choices.

However, it is not always evident that morally problematic behavior results from deliberate choices. Usually, people's everyday actions focus only on avoiding condemnation. We try to protect our moral self-image and maintain a sense of being an ethical person.

Complex behavioral disorders indicate that moral health relies on self-awareness, self-evaluation, and self-restraint. Researchers highlight that immoral behavior is challenging because it often occurs outside of our awareness or conscious control. They demonstrate that immoral actions are associated with brain processes involving increased cognitive conflict and shifts in perceptual attention.[18]

It is the tendency toward a purposeful and objective moral self that

---

[17] Tangeny JP, et.al. <u>Moral Emotions and Moral Behavior</u>. Annu Rev Psychol (Vol 58), 2007
[18] Cosmides, L. et.al. <u>Detecting Cheaters</u>. Trends Cogn Sci. (Vol. 9), 2005

mainly develops people's moral capacities for moral health. The process of growing in moral health is rooted in individuals' moral selves. It is a person's proper and well-developed moral self that promotes growth in moral health.

Generally, moral human nature is often expressed with normative intent or at least practiced with normative results. However, evolutionary science, neuroscience, and health sciences emphasize that humans share a moral nature similar to their physical nature.

Scientists assert that moral human nature is a biological trait because the human brain is wired to predetermine behaviors. To address the moral health issues of our time, the traditional methods provided by society and culture for cultivating a moral self need refinement to enhance the moral sense that develops a moral self capable of cultivating behaviors that meet today's challenges.

Health science researchers show that behaviors cause various effects, intricately and profoundly influencing the interconnected system of mind, body, and spirit aspects of human health. Neuroscience emphasizes that there is significant brain plasticity, which enables behavioral change and can contribute to the development of moral health in individuals.

Neurologically and behaviorally, humans are highly adaptable through learning, unmatched by other organisms. The health sciences suggest that modifying mental and psychological factors can reasonably enhance one's moral sense and moral self, leading to positive behavioral outcomes. There is an essential need for the educational, health, and legal systems to consider an individual's moral sense and moral self in human development.

Nature always follows its course in all human growth and development. It becomes evident when we consider how we must constantly change for self-improvement. This can also be seen through the evolving moral sense and moral self in our times. There are many signs that we are naturally evolving in a moral consciousness that surpasses the rules and expectations of traditional moral life.

Experts in human consciousness studies maintain that natural evolution is an ongoing process. They argue it continues today through the development of humanity's new consciousness. They assert it is pre-ordained by the evolutionary process of the natural order. It is believed that the problems and challenges humanity faces today are connected to the evolution of our moral consciousness.

The moral health of individuals is rooted in a moral self that reflects evolved human consciousness, not just in superficial moral norms and ideals. When people focus only on moral rules, principles, and cultural ideals, the results are apparent. Their daily actions often bypass legal requirements, ethical standards, and moral instructions.

In conclusion, there is a consensus in modern science that moral health is developed through brain processes involving abstract cognitive abilities that regulate negative phylogenetic instincts. Human intellectual, emotional, and moral capacities are crucial in maintaining moral health. It must be recognized that moral health is an essential part of overall health, comparable to physical and mental health. Moral health is part of the same cause-and-effect framework as other aspects of nature. It is an existential phenomenon and an intrinsic aspect of human existence. Scientific insights into human moral nature have underscored the importance of moral health as a crucial component of overall well-being and a key pathway to the well-being of humanity.

WHAT IS MORAL HEALTH

The dictionary defines health as "the condition of an organism or one of its parts in which it performs its vital functions normally or properly." Historically, hospital, medical, and clinical services have focused on diagnosing and treating to restore and maintain health, not on preventing sickness and disease. People's general understanding of health is limited to the physical and/or psycho-emotional aspects of well-being. In our world, health is usually the last concern until it is lost. Healthcare often does not receive the importance it deserves.

The World Health Organization defines health as "a state of complete physical, mental, and social well-being and not merely the absence of disease or infirmity." Although the moral and spiritual aspects are core human experiences, the official definition of health does not emphasize the importance of moral and spiritual health. Typically, the goal of health care does not include addressing moral and spiritual well-being.

From ancient times to the pre-modern era, the approach to health has focused on the whole person rather than just illness or specific body parts. However, today, globally, there has been a significant shift from diagnosing and treating disease to promoting and setting standards of health that include moral, spiritual, social, and environmental aspects. A holistic approach now emphasizes the entire person—mind, body, and spirit—in treatment and healthcare.

Holistic health might seem like a modern idea, but it isn't. Historically, there has been a focus on holistic health, an approach that has endured for thousands of years. The connection between moral health and holistic health also has a long history. Ayurveda, one of the world's oldest medical systems, emphasizes moral health by stressing that good health is maintained through a way of life focused on higher goals. Dharma (correct behavior) across all areas of life was the foundation of ancient Indian society and played a key role in good health. Dharma highlights that good health involves both the spiritual and moral aspects of human nature.

Chinese medicine is another of the world's oldest medical systems. According to the Huangdi Neijing, good health is viewed as the result of emotional balance and effective adaptation to the environment. The ancient Chinese idea of health was not just the absence of symptoms but the presence of an intense vital energy, known as qi. Qi was believed to promote inner balance and harmony, which are fundamental to moral health, and they enhance overall well-being.

The ancient Greeks developed the physiocratic school of thought, maintaining that good health cannot be separated from the environment or human behavior. They recognized that moral values are just as important as the mind and body and are an essential part of human nature. Socrates believed no harm could be done to a moral person because the soul surpasses even the struggles of mental disorders. In The Republic, Plato suggested that a healthy individual practices the cardinal virtues: prudence in making judgments, courage in facing dangers, temperance in controlling appetites, and justice in demonstrating inner harmony through disinterested good conduct. For Plato, moral suffering was not just a metaphor, and he argued that failing in moral duties significantly impacts health.

For centuries, moral philosophers, religious scholars, legal scholars, and political scientists have explored abstract moral principles that govern moral thinking, feelings, and actions, shaping how individuals interact within society. Their efforts focused on whether specific behaviors align with various moral ideals. However, it was modern psychology's interest in behavior—motivated by developmental questions and clinical implications of moral issues—that shifted the focus of contemporary sciences toward understanding moral phenomena as connected to health. This psychological perspective on moral behaviors led to research into the neurobiological mechanisms of moral thinking, emotion, and behavior. It inspired efforts to investigate the underlying processes of moral well-being empirically.

The concept of moral health stems from real evidence of "moral suffering." It is often experienced as internal chaos, emotional pain, and an unstable sense of self. It manifests through self-sabotaging behaviors caused by shame, guilt, fear, anger, despair, and other negative emotions. The idea of "moral suffering" was developed from research on combat trauma.[19] In those studies, it was described as severe emotional and social trauma endured on the battlefield. This highlights a kind of "inner psyche mess," with emotional stress that harms a person's health and overall well-being.

As humans, at some point, we all experience moral suffering and moral distress. Scientific literature shows that poor moral health can be recognized through people's experience of "moral suffering." Moral suffering typically manifests as a loss of personal equilibrium and homeostasis. Health professionals believe that there are different levels of moral suffering in individuals dealing with physical and mental health issues.

People burdened by moral suffering report symptoms similar to those experienced by morally injured combat veterans. Moral suffering involves intense psycho-emotional distress, psychosocial trauma, or psychospiritual pain resulting from morally wrong acts for which one feels responsible. The effects of moral suffering permeate daily life across various settings, including work,

---

[19] Drescher et al. An Exploration of the Viability and Usefulness of the Construct of Moral Injury in War Veterans. Traumatology (Vol 17), 2011

home, and society. These symptoms range from mild, like moodiness, impatience, and lack of empathy, to subclinical issues like sleep disturbances, tantrums, bullying, binge eating or drinking, and physical symptoms like headaches, asthma, and hypertension.[20]

In daily life, moral suffering is an individual's experience of profound psycho-emotional stress that can be hard to express. Individuals who experience moral suffering may exhibit physical signs of stress and a disruption to their psychological well-being. It can manifest through uncontrolled self-sabotaging behaviors. Moral suffering happens when individuals act in ways that are self-destructive and violate or undermine the common good and higher principles in life. Often, it is an unnoticed self-damaging process within the person because moral suffering is not recognized as a health concern. Frequently, it is denied or hidden deep in the mind.

How can we define moral health? Describing moral health as a health concept can be somewhat elusive. There is no clear definition of moral health in scientific literature. What can be said is that moral health is an emerging science that goes beyond abstract philosophical ideas of morality. Health scientists and researchers view growing moral health as the development of cognitions and emotions that guide behavioral patterns toward an admirable and lifelong pursuit of becoming a better and healthier version of oneself, emphasizing other-orientedness and the common good.

Although there is no clear definition of moral health in the health sciences, the scientific literature describes it as the development of innate emotional, cognitive, and behavioral abilities that foster moral capacities aligned with higher purposes and ideals, such as truth, fairness, and justice. It involves advanced cognitive functions, such as perception, insight, intuition, and practical wisdom, which enable humans to flourish as individual yet interdependent social beings. It also reflects a person's capacity to morally adapt

---

[20] Jinkerson,JD. Defining and assessing moral injury: A syndrome perspective. Traumatology (Vol. 22) 2016

when facing vulnerable and challenging environments filled with uncertainty and risk.

Moral health is much more complex and multifaceted than the standard view that it simply means following traditional morality. In modern health sciences, human physiology, biochemistry, cognition, emotion, and socialization are seen as interconnected aspects of moral health. Neuroscience reveals that humans possess a moral biology that provides the organic framework necessary to develop and nurture moral health, much like physical health. Neuroscientists emphasize that this moral biology is essential for creating a functional moral capacity. Additionally, neuroscientific evidence demonstrates that human intellectual functions make humans' moral nature distinct within the animal kingdom.

Modern sciences provide evidence that moral health is an essential, experiential aspect of well-being. They emphasize the positive experience of moral health as a state of feeling deeply secure, socially transparent, and invigorating in all life situations. Scientists and researchers view moral health as rooted in inherent human abilities, such as self-awareness, empathy, intuition, and perception. It reflects the human moral nature through the potential to nurture mutuality, trust, integrity, respect, dignity, and other distinctly human qualities.

In the clinical literature, physical and mental health, as well as illness and disease, are clearly defined. The assessment of physical pain, suffering, and disorder is based on rigorous clinical studies. There are established diagnostic criteria for evaluating symptoms of physical illness and disease. Similarly, mental health is defined, and psychological and social diagnostic metrics exist to identify mental health issues. However, there are no standardized diagnostic criteria for moral health, and it is only vaguely defined within clinical health literature.

However, growing evidence suggests that moral suffering poses a significant threat to overall health and well-being.[21] It negatively affects the human psyche by stemming from underlying feelings of guilt, shame, self-blame, and self-hate. This causes psycho-emotional wounds that impact neuroendocrine and immune system complexities, seriously harming health. When we experience moral suffering, it disrupts the balance of the human psyche, leading to neurobiological imbalances that underlie physical and mental health problems. Daily, people's subtle moral pain and suffering negatively influence brain chemistry and affect homeostasis.

All human suffering relates to one or more components of health. The typical experience of poor health involves some form of suffering, and moral suffering often goes unnoticed by us. Moral suffering reflects the negative experience of moral health. As a health-related issue, moral pain and suffering are no different from physical or mental pain and suffering.

Good health is linked to the moral and spiritual aspects—core components of human nature—and is always reflected in our daily relationships, behaviors, and lifestyles. Poor moral health involves cognitive and behavioral abilities that are unsustainable because they cause moral suffering. Usually, we overlook the impact of our moral reasoning, which underpins our moral pain and suffering. The way we live, treat ourselves, and treat others is all connected to moral health. Immoral behaviors not only lead to punishment by the justice system but also produce punitive effects on brain chemistry that harm personal well-being and health.

Recently, neuroscience's growing interest in human moral nature has expanded our understanding of the cognitive and emotional processes behind moral motivations, decisions, and behaviors, as well as their neural bases. It has also revealed insights into the neurology of abnormal moral behavior. The evidence shows that moral human nature is one of the most sophisticated aspects of our species, essential for developing moral health and leading a better

---

[21] Epstein E.G., Hamric A.B. Moral distress, moral residue, and the crescendo effect. J. Clin. Ethics. (Vol 20); 2009

human life.

Neuroscience shows that the neural basis of developing moral health depends on the brain mechanisms responsible for higher intellectual functions. The brain provides consciousness, which is fundamental to human nature and essential for developing moral health. Neuroscience researchers highlight the brain's ability to create moral capacities. They point to the neurobiological processes involved in cultivating moral health across all aspects of well-being.

Humans possess an essential organic moral system that predisposes us to moral reasoning and motivation, leading to behaviors that promote moral health. What neuroscience is showing today is an innate "moral biology" that allows us to go beyond the moral rules of conventional morality.

Moral health is a complex phenomenon involving interconnected intrapersonal and interpersonal systems rooted in human nature that make humans uniquely moral beings. Nowadays, neuroscience is uncovering the brain mechanisms and processes behind the moral self, helping us create better standards of moral health than traditional ideals and principles of morality.

What is known so far is that the human biological capacity for moral health involves the precisely tuned brain structures and neurochemistry responsible for awareness, judgment, motivation, and behavior. The natural human abilities of intuition, cognition, and emotion are vital to developing moral health. Environmental influences also play a crucial role in shaping and maintaining moral well-being. Scientific evidence suggests that ethical, moral, and legal codes are unlikely to be effective in promoting the positive development of moral health.[22]

There is a growing interest among health researchers to demonstrate that moral health is most influential on a person's physical, mental, and social well-being. It helps us recognize and validate human moral capacities as fundamental to human nature and crucial for health improvement.

---

[22] Noam GG & Wren TE (Eds.) The moral self. MIT Press (1993).

Neuroscience findings show that human moral nature involves cognitions and emotions that influence behaviors affecting people's daily health and well-being.

There are inherent elements of a complete, indivisible human organism that give us flexible, adaptable moral abilities that can't be reduced to a set of moral principles, codes, and standards. Recent neuroscientific evidence suggests that humans are wired to understand and experience the world in rational and deliberative ways, revealing what is moral in human nature.[23] The intuitive, emotional, and relational aspects of human moral nature enable human life to differ significantly from that of animals. This helps us today to distinguish between traditional morality and the scientific idea of moral health.

Differentiating the Concept of Morality and Moral Health

Today, we face many human problems rooted in people's moral health. A quick look at the daily news shows this clearly. Issues like economic inequality, dehumanizing poverty, violence, heinous crimes, social unrest, geopolitical tensions, wars, and even climate change all involve our moral well-being. Moreover, health experts emphasize that the physical and mental health problems overwhelming hospitals, mental institutions, and prisons often have underlying moral health issues.

Most people consider being moral as a key part of who they are. As part of their identity, they want to be perceived as moral. Usually, everyone likes to think they are moral. However, this is not always true; often, we pretend to be moral. Many even believe they are somewhat more moral than others and find examples of "good" behaviors to support this idea. Researchers in behavioral ethics have demonstrated that people employ various justification mechanisms that enable them to act wrongfully and still feel morally justified.[24]

How would one describe a moral person? According to the legal system, the individual is law-abiding. In the religious system, the individual is right with God. For the mental health system, the person is socially well-

---

[23] Gazzaniga, M. S. The social brain: Discovering the networks of the mind. Basic Books (1985).
[24] Shalvi et al. Self-Serving Justifications: Doing Wrong and Feeling Moral. APS (Vol 24) 2015

adjusted. To family and friends, one is simply a good and decent person. In contrast, people judged as immoral or perceived as depraved are described as criminal, deviant, pathological, sinful, or evil.

But these are superficial perceptions. An incorrect and incomplete understanding of what it means to be a moral person, along with a lack of proper grasp of moral health, has resulted in a multitude of selfish and powerful individuals on the world stage. At the same time, throughout history, we have known people who have broken prescribed moral standards from a position of moral strength. Through personal integrity and character, they demonstrated a different sense of moral self-identity. They were seen as distinct by aligning with higher ideals and purposes. People admire them as moral icons for their luminous lives.

When addressing moral issues, we typically think in terms of morality rather than moral health. As a concept, morality helps us differentiate between intentions, decisions, and actions to identify those that are proper (right) from those that are improper (wrong). Conventional morality is a set of standards or principles derived from a code of conduct based on a particular philosophy, religion, or culture, or it may come from a standard that an individual believes should be universal. In the literature on conventional morality, whether in ethics, moral philosophy, or jurisprudence, there is no universal term for moral suffering. One reason for this is that morality is described in abstract terms, not as a health-related phenomenon.

Rather than focusing on developing their moral health, people often engage in conventional morality because it seems more relevant to life. The main reason is that it helps them appear as moral individuals. The moral ideals or virtues of traditional morality are used to present a socially acceptable moral persona, protect their public image, and enhance it. However, in everyday life, moral standards and norms can also be bypassed to serve self-interest, ego, and self-centered goals. Social Psychology researchers emphasize that conventional morality functions as a social mechanism to maintain a favorable self-image and social reputation. They note that people often see themselves as moral, even when they recognize that their actions do not align with their stated moral ideals and principles.[25]

What social scientists and researchers reveal is that often the ideals and principles of conventional morality do not effectively restrain behaviors that harm moral health. Morality shapes the moral self, which influences people's cognitive and emotional processes and guides daily behaviors in the moral domain. However, even a strong commitment to morality doesn't stop individuals from abandoning harmful behaviors. The moral self remains unquestioned and unchallenged. All our everyday actions and behaviors affecting moral health are rooted in a rigid, flawed, and corrupt moral self. Regular encounters with hypocrites, fraudsters, sociopaths, psychopaths, or criminals highlight the failure of conventional morality to promote moral health. We may act habitually "morally" without experiencing "moral health."

Everyone chooses a life orientation somewhere along a spectrum between self-centeredness and other-centeredness; no one is entirely on one side or the other. Naturally, we all begin with an instinct for self-preservation, but persistent self-centeredness that prevents a deeper self-understanding leads to different behavioral outcomes than when it does not. The well-developed moral self is essentially other-centered, yet also self-aware. It manifests in care and concern for both oneself and others. As people grow in moral maturity, they tend to emphasize behaviors that foster inclusiveness and interconnectedness. When a person's moral self does not prevent self-centeredness, their ability to exhibit behaviors that promote moral health is diminished.

Self-exploration is a fundamental aspect of human nature driven by our

---

[25] Bandura A. Moral disengagement in the perpetration of inhumanities. Personality and Social Psychology Review 3. (1999).

Bandura A. Moral disengagement in the perpetration of inhumanities. Personality and Social Psychology Review 3. (1999).

moral instincts. It involves intrapersonal and interpersonal self-understanding. Although it may seem unnatural and challenging, understanding and appreciating others' perspectives, values, and behaviors in daily life is crucial for developing moral health. Recent findings in health sciences indicate that a focus on others in our life orientation is essential for moral growth. This is because adopting an other-centered approach depends on neural networks involved in higher cognitive functions, which develop abilities such as self-awareness, self-evaluation, and self-regulation.

Being connected to the world is essential for anyone genuinely committed to moral health. By recognizing interdependence as crucial for human life and well-being, a person can take actions based on a stronger sense of moral duty towards everyone. When people acknowledge and utilize the strengths within their moral nature, they develop a self-identity and way of life that are free from self-centeredness. This helps reduce self-delusions, behavioral inconsistencies, and moral contradictions. The moral motivation behind actions remains unaffected by social structures and competition.

Typically, there is no single clear definition of moral health in society or culture. For most people, moral health is a relative concept that depends on various parameters. For example, the social norms in a society might be parameters to develop moral health, but not in another, or what is considered moral at one time and place may be immoral at another. When ordinary people make moral choices and decisions, they do so based on the moral reasoning shaped by a society's moral framework and conventional morality.

Thus, for most of us, "moral knowledge" consists of codified and prescribed moral ideals, principles, and values taught through behavioral training and habituation. This black-and-white view of morality overlooks the biological and emotional aspects of humans, as well as the mental processes involved in developing moral health. The vital role of the human brain in forming moral understanding and motivating actions that promote moral well-being is often overlooked. In short, life's focus is not on the higher level of personhood, which supports the psychosocial maturity of individuals.

When the focus is solely on conventional morality, we often concentrate only on appearing moral rather than fostering moral health. We want others to see us as "decent," "good," and moral. We adopt the moral self to avoid judgment and condemnation, even when we fail to meet the expected moral standards. In practicing conventional morality, people are often driven to protect their public image rather than develop genuine moral health. This occurs even if conventional morality hinders the growth of a mature, more relevant moral self, which is needed to address pressing moral issues, resolve dilemmas, and engage with real-life moral challenges.

The concept of moral health has been part of human culture for ages. For thousands of years, religion and law have guided people's moral reasoning and actions. However, we know that dishonest individuals have often used religion and law to justify wrongdoings. Even today, evidence shows that moral hypocrites, who are strictly moral or legalistic, usually ignore genuine ethical, moral, and legal standards. Despite following traditional morality, people frequently act in ways that harm moral health. When it comes to improving moral health, the moral phenomenon exists outside of religion and law. Moral human nature existed before culture, religion, and law, and it surpasses them.

Ordinary people's everyday sense of moral health refers to the set of standards for acceptable behaviors. We think in moral terms to gain approval for our actions. From infancy, we go through 'conscience formation,' which guides our daily moral thinking, feelings, and actions. We live with a moral conscience that judges us as good or bad, right or wrong, and it is also used to judge others. When someone intentionally violates moral standards, even while knowing right from wrong, we see that person as immoral. If someone is unaffected by moral standards, we consider that individual non-moral, and they are regarded as amoral if they are not concerned with morality, while still recognizing the difference between right and wrong.

The limit of moral conscience is that, generally, we do not always recognize that actions and behaviors favorable to cultivating moral health often require abandoning short-term interests to achieve long-term benefits or being willing to sacrifice oneself for higher purposes and the common good in human life. This conception of moral health often involves going beyond established moral standards of conscience and social mores, or even crossing them. The concept of moral health is not just about distinguishing right from wrong and good from destructive or prosocial behaviors.

The moral self is the tool through which moral health is developed. One can think of the moral self as the 'ground of one's being.' It is essential to human existence. The idea of one's moral self relates more to moral health than to merely following moral standards. The statement that "good people can do bad things" shows that to understand moral health, we need to look at the deeper roots of deviant or harmful behaviors. Harmful actions are not solely the result of breaking moral norms and rules. Every day, people act with flawed moral reasoning and a misunderstood concept of the moral self, which harms their moral health. They are limited by moral reasoning based on external standards rather than internalized ones.

Some may think that the legal and criminal systems are connected to moral health. However, this idea seems far-fetched, considering the current moral climate in our world. The moral aspect of human health is embedded in the fabric of the natural world. It isn't just an addition created by culture, religion, and society.

The accurate measure of moral health in a person comes from internalized standards. It involves moral consciousness, not moral conscience, which is based on moral standards. Conventional morality's ideals and standards do not limit the cognitions and behaviors that result from moral consciousness. Moral consciousness encourages cognitive processes that respond positively to every urgent issue in the moral sphere. It clarifies the immediate moral dilemma and conflict, helping to resolve any moral situation. The moral sense and motivation for actions go beyond the pressures and demands of moral conscience.

Moral health relies on more advanced cognitive skills, such as prudence, self-reflection, and self-regulation. The development of emotional and mental abilities, such as truth-seeking and higher-minded thinking for greater life purposes, helps form a more mature moral self, which supports the cultivation of moral health. As people develop moral health, they grow in their capacity to experience awe and wonder, unity and love, transcendence and wholeness, altruism and gratitude, as well as serenity and peace. In individuals who advance in moral consciousness, we observe a moral motivation that differs from conventional morality. These individuals exhibit behaviors of empathetic amiability, interdependence, altruism, and cooperation for the common good and the greater good. They are the symbols of moral health in our era.

To promote moral health, we must recognize it as a natural part of the world and vital to overall well-being. Moral health is part of the same cause-and-effect system as other natural phenomena. It involves thoughts and actions directed toward others. Human behavior is as much a part of nature as the human body. In the animal kingdom, behaviors are inherent to each species. The ideas of good and bad behaviors should not be seen as fixed ideals or absolutes but rather in terms of their effects on oneself and others. Similar to toxins in air, food, or water, unhealthy behaviors act as toxins that harm a person's well-being. Human actions follow natural cause-and-effect patterns concerning moral health. Just as nutrients, exercise, and sleep influence physical and mental health, daily behaviors profoundly affect moral health and overall well-being.

The moral health of people is far more complex and multifaceted than most realize. The proper functioning of the human body relies on physiology, biochemistry, cognitive, neurological, and social systems that are innate, interconnected, and interdependent. It is not governed solely by prescriptions and ideals. Humans naturally have the adaptable abilities necessary to develop moral health, which cannot be reduced to a mere collection of moral norms, codes, or social institutions. Moral health is an ongoing, dynamic process that involves physiological, biochemical, cognitive, emotional, behavioral, and social development. It influences human experience but cannot be fully defined by traditional notions of morality.

The concept of moral health has a positive impact across various health-related areas, shifting the focus from negative behavioral issues to life guidance and holistic health-promoting choices. Practically, it provides a helpful framework for creating preventive and protective measures to address the inevitable moral and ethical vulnerabilities. The concept of moral health offers a constructive tool for understanding and regulating daily actions, as well as managing the challenges of moral subjectivity and moral suffering that arise in people's daily lives.

The lowest level of moral health is marked by a severe lack of empathy or emotional depth, no genuine remorse for antisocial actions, and a tendency toward instrumental aggression. Scientific evidence of this psycho-emotional state exists not only in sociopaths, psychopaths, and criminals, whether proven or not, but also in "decent" people in society. The behaviors of such individuals demonstrate a callous, manipulative, and arrogant temperament in their personality functioning within society.

Neuroscientists have found that psychopathic individuals show abnormal brain structure.[26] The brain regions involved with assessing, learning, and empathetic connection do not function normally. This evidence suggests that, in many practical ways, improving moral health in daily life will always depend on people's ability to assess and learn. The brain mechanisms responsible for evaluating and learning from experiences are crucial to developing better empathy, a positive indicator of moral health, and essential for cultivating it.

---

[26] Hare, RD, et. al. Psychopathy and the DSM-IV criteria for antisocial personality disorder. Journal of Abnormal Psychology 100(3) (1991).

Moral health relates to everyday human activity, positively influencing overall health from within. As part of the natural order, moral human nature is outward-focused and heavily other-oriented. It develops from specific behaviors, like altruism, that consistently benefit a person's overall health.

Moral health is as personal as it is collective. Behaviors have consequences not only for the individual but also for others. To foster moral health, daily actions should focus on self-improvement, being other-oriented, and building a healthier humanity. Moral health aims to realize full human potential, making individuals the agents of humanity's moral well-being.

THE NEUROSCIENCE OF MORAL HEALTH

The discussion about our innate human moral capacities dates back thousands of years. Since then, it has mainly been debated in philosophy, theology, law, and psychology. For a long time, the human moral phenomenon was only viewed through abstract ideas and ideals, without scientific investigation. The idea of studying it empirically was not proposed until recent times. Today, scientists show that the human brain is wired for moral reasoning, moral emotion, and moral behavior. They reveal that humans possess unique moral abilities not found in other animals. They provide evidence of a "moral brain," a neural network that can help us develop moral health.

Biology and neuroscience have challenged philosophical debates on morality by revealing physiological and genetic factors that underlie the moral capacities unique to humans. Neuroscience, neurobiology, and neuropsychology are sciences that help us better understand the functional and clinical neuroanatomy behind this vital aspect of human health. Scientists and researchers have created the exciting possibility of supplementing abstract philosophical ideas with empirical science to better understand moral health.

What we are learning from scientific evidence is that moral reasoning and moral emotion are among the most sophisticated features of the human mind, and that moral behavior results from a complex process that, although influenced by genes and environment, is ultimately controlled by the brain. Neuroscience reveals that specific brain areas are involved in both normal and abnormal behaviors, affecting individuals' moral health levels. The significant advances in neuroscience are helping us understand the neural basis of moral health.

Is there a neurological basis for moral health and/or moral disease? We will answer this question by examining (1) the historical development of the clinical study of moral behavior, (2) the clinical neuroanatomy of the "moral brain," (3) the clinical neuroanatomy of moral behavior, (4) the clinical neuroanatomy of the moral self, and (5) the clinical neuroanatomy of moral health and moral disease.

History of the Clinical Study of Moral Behavior

Over the past two centuries, a growing body of empirical evidence has emerged to understand the neurological origins of moral behavior better. Cesare Lombroso, an Italian physician, was the first to attempt to study sociopathy empirically. He developed an anthropological theory of delinquency through five editions of his "L'uomo Delinquente" (The Delinquent Man).[27] After measuring the shape and size of several criminals' heads, he concluded that the somatic traits characteristic of these individuals resembled those of primitive humans and that their antisocial tendencies were present at birth, making them hereditary. He implied that brain functions and genetics influence issues related to moral health.

But long before Lombroso, in 1806, Philippe Pinel, a French psychiatrist, introduced the term "manie sans delire" (mania without delusion) to describe a condition marked by cruel behaviors without affecting cognition, perception, or memory.[28] An American doctor, Benjamin Rush, also described

---

[27] Lombroso, C. The criminal man, studies in relation to anthropology, forensic medicine, and prison disciplines. Ulrico Hoepli, 1876
[28] Pinel, P. Medical-philosophical treatise on mental alienation or mania. Brosson, 1801

a similar condition, which he called "moral derangement," in his work, "Medical Inquiries and Diseases of the Mind."[29]

Similar to Pinel's observations, Rush identified the antisocial traits of individuals who exhibited no remorse, guilt, or concern about the negative consequences of their actions. Later, these behaviors were called sociopathic and psychopathic. In addition to clinical observations, data from ethological studies on complex social behaviors in animals helped interpret many aspects of human behavior from an evolutionary perspective.

This line of inquiry has grown from the idea that human moral nature is connected to the evolution of the human brain. Evolutionary anthropologists demonstrate that brain mechanisms have evolved to support cognitive abilities that foster behaviors essential for human survival.[30] They highlight the human brain's ability to develop moral reasoning, which has evolved in tandem with other brain mechanisms that have advanced throughout human evolution.

In modern times, understanding the neurobiological basis of moral health is supported by observations of patients who experience sudden changes in their social interactions due to cerebral lesions, as well as studies on normal and pathological behaviors using neuroimaging techniques. The available research indicates that a neural network is involved in behaviors related to a person's level of moral health.[31] Specifically, this neural network is connected to the ventromedial prefrontal cortex and its multiple links to the limbic lobe, thalamus, and brainstem.

In recent decades, behavioral and neuroscientific studies of the moral phenomenon of humans have grown in volume and complexity. Some of the clinical fields investigating moral aptitude, moral reasoning, and moral

---

[29] Rush B. Medical Inquiries and Observations, Upon the Diseases of the Mind. Kimber & Richardson (1812).

[30] Lorenz, K. Evolution and modification of behavior. The University of Chicago Press (1986)

[31] Damasio AR, Tranel D, Damasio H. Individuals with sociopathic behavior caused by frontal damage fail to respond autonomically to social stimuli. Behav Brain Res. 41,(1990)

Batts S, Brain lesions and their implications in criminal responsibility. Behav Sci Law, 27 (2009)

behavior—the levels of moral health in people—include clinical neurology and psychiatry, psychoneuroendocrinology, neuroimaging, neurophysiology, neuropathology, and behavioral genetics. Advances in clinical neurology, psychoneuroendocrinology, and psychiatry have generated a wealth of knowledge that can help us address current issues of moral health.

The Neuroanatomy of the 'Moral Brain': An Overview

In recent decades, neuroscientists have discussed a "moral brain" that underpins behaviors influencing a person's moral health. They have not pinpointed a specific brain region associated with the "moral brain." The human brain does not have a single center responsible for moral health. Instead, the "moral brain" is made up of multiple regions and circuits related to emotion, planning, problem-solving, empathy, and prosocial behavior, which work together to support moral development.[32]

To understand the neurobiological basis of moral health, it is necessary to examine the various neural systems and brain mechanisms that influence daily thinking, emotions, motivation, and behavior. We must understand how neural systems work together to produce moral reasoning, moral emotions, and moral actions, all of which impact moral health. The functional and clinical neuroanatomy of moral human nature underscores the complexity and the multiple neural controls involved in moral capacities.[33]

Scientists have demonstrated that an extensive functional neural network, often called the "moral brain," influences moral health. This network includes both cortical and subcortical structures. These structures include the medial frontal cortex (mPFC) for understanding mental states and thoughts, the amygdala for emotional reactions, the ventromedial frontal cortex (vmPFC) for integrating thoughts and emotions in decision-making and prosocial

---

[32] Greene, J D & Paxton, J M. Patterns of neural activity associated with honest and dishonest moral decisions. Proceedings of the National Academy of Sciences, Vol. 106, (2009).
[33] Raine A, Yang Y. Neural foundations to moral reasoning and antisocial behavior. Soc Cogn Affect Neurosc. Vol 1 (2006)

behaviors, the dorsolateral prefrontal cortex (dlPFC) for self-control and intelligence, the insula for body awareness, and the posterior superior temporal sulcus (pSTS) for understanding others' intentions.[34]

Other brain regions involved in a person's moral abilities are the anterior cingulate cortex, which mediates the 'conflict' between emotional and rational components of moral sense, and the posterior cingulate cortex, which is more closely associated with emotion and social skills.

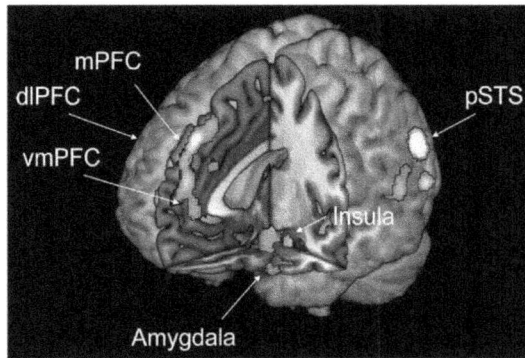

Creative Commons Public Domain

Neuroscience has improved our understanding of not only the cognitive and emotional processes involved in a person's moral abilities but also the brain structures underlying them. Among the brain regions, the frontal, temporal, and cingulate cortices are involved in an individual's moral processing.

The neuroscience of moral health shows that when people do moral tasks, the normal activity of the brain's neuromoral network follows specific patterns. In short, the ventromedial prefrontal cortex is the central part of the neuro-moral circuit, helping process morally charged stimuli and produce states like empathy, charity, fairness, and their opposites, such as impropriety, dishonesty, cruelty, and others. The dorsolateral prefrontal cortex helps integrate these states, supports moral reasoning, and enables individuals to

---

[34] Greene JD, et.al. The neural bases of cognitive conflict and control in moral judgment. Neuron, vol.44 (2004)

control or ignore emotional states that may compromise moral behavior. The orbitofrontal cortex is involved in recognizing and responding to moral or immoral actions by others, enabling the mapping and imitation of observed behaviors. The amygdala detects sensory emotional stimuli that haven't been integrated yet and sends them to the ventromedial prefrontal cortex for moral assessment and processing. The mesolimbic reward pathway is linked to feelings of pleasure when performing a non-moral act toward a hostile individual. The cingulate cortex helps manage conflicts during immoral actions and is associated with feelings of envy when others overtake individuals.[35]

The diagram shows possible circuits of the "moral brain," with the ventromedial prefrontal cortex as the main integrating center connected to other cortical, limbic, hypothalamic, and brainstem areas.

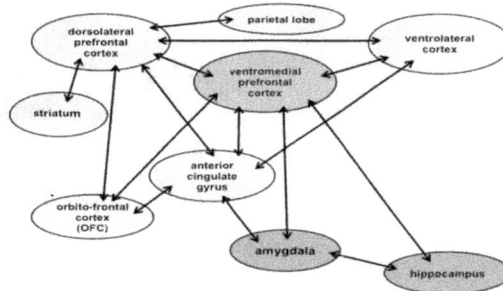

Creative Commons Public Domain

The "moral brain" shares neural structures that also govern thinking, feeling, and behavior in areas beyond moral issues. Because moral reasoning and behavior are complex, some of these brain structures share circuits with those controlling other processes, such as emotions.

In addition to brain regions, brain chemicals known as neuromodulators also influence an individual's moral emotions, thereby affecting moral behavior. These chemicals modify neuronal activity, excitability,

---

[35]Pascual L, Rodrigues P, Gallardo-Pujol D, How Morality Works in the Brain: A Functional and Structural Perspective of Moral Behavior. Integr. Neurosci. September 2013
Moll J, de Oliveira-Souza R, Eslinger PJ, Morals and the human brain: a working model. Neuroreport. March 2003

and synaptic functions, which are involved in a person's behavioral tendencies. In daily life, we observe that moral emotions and moral behavior are varied and dynamic. They differ between individuals and within the same individual over time. This highlights the importance of neuromodulators in creating moral emotions and shaping moral behaviors.

Several chemicals produced in the brain influence moral emotions, impacting behaviors related to moral health and disease. The neuromodulator oxytocin has garnered significant attention and is often referred to as the "moral molecule." Oxytocin can increase trust and generosity in some situations but may also heighten envy and bias in others. From an evolutionary perspective, it is a primal molecule found across mammalian species, playing a key role in the mother-child relationship by enhancing bonding and reducing fear and anxiety.

Another neuromodulator, serotonin, plays a significant role in social behaviors, particularly aggression, and is produced in both the brain and the gastrointestinal tract.[36] Brain studies show that the highest levels of serotonin are found in various limbic structures, such as the cingulate, entorhinal, insular, and temporopolar regions, as well as in the ventral and pallidal parts of the striatum and the medial orbitofrontal cortex. Serotonin has been shown to influence moral judgment by increasing negative feelings when we see others in harm. It affects human concerns for harm and fairness. The aversion to harm gives moral sense to promote the greater good. One challenge for researchers is understanding how serotonin influences the complexity of both moral emotion and moral behavior.

Additionally, the complex and multifaceted neural control of moral health involves the roles of genes and hormones and is part of several neurobiological functional regions. It is now commonly believed that genetic alterations and abnormalities in brain function can be linked to criminal behavior. Geneticists suggest that complex behavioral disorders can be partly

---

[36] Way BM, et al. Architectonic distribution of the serotonin transporter within the orbitofrontal cortex of the vervet monkey. Neuroscience, IBRO. September (2007)

attributed to variations in DNA sequences and environmental factors. Researchers have found that both genetic and environmental influences play significant roles in the development of psychopathy.[37]

Furthermore, researchers indicate that social and emotional processing has a strong reciprocal connection with the endocrine system.[38] Along with genetic factors, hormones are known to profoundly influence cognition and behavior by interfering with brain metabolism and neuronal function. Clinical studies reveal that lower levels of the hormone cortisol limit empathy and guilt, explaining the constricted emotionality that characterizes antisocial disorder and psychopathic behaviors. Another hormone involved in aggressive behavior is testosterone. High testosterone levels enhance attention to aggressive stimuli, downregulate the interaction between cognitive and emotional brain systems, and are associated with dominant aggressive behavior.[39]

During moral decision-making, individuals with high testosterone levels are more inclined to make utilitarian choices, particularly when such choices involve acts of aggression and harm to others. The hormonal indicator of violence is the testosterone/cortisol ratio. When high testosterone combines with low cortisol, aggression becomes unchecked, and the individual could pose a danger to others.

Modern-day sciences, such as neuroscience, neurobiology, and neuropsychology reveal that genetic, endocrine, environmental, and cultural factors influence behaviors that affect one's moral health. The scientific evidence on the function of the neuro-moral circuit reveals how brain regions and circuits influence the development of moral health. The mechanistic understanding of the moral phenomenon in human nature greatly demystifies

---

[37] Gunter TD, et.al. Behavioral genetics in antisocial spectrum disorders and psychopathy: a review of the recent literature. Behav Sci Law vol 28 (2010)

[38] Terburg D, et.al. The testosterone-cortisol ratio: a hormonal marker for proneness to social aggression. Int J Law Psychiatry, vol 32. (2009)

[39] Terburg D, et.al. The testosterone-cortisol ratio: a hormonal marker for proneness to social aggression. Int J Law Psychiatry, vol 32. (2009)

traditional assumptions of conventional morality. It challenges the collective interpretation of what it means to be human, with significant implications for law, public policy, and moral well-being.

The Clinical Neuroanatomy of Moral Behavior

Moral behavior relies on the brain's mechanisms for representing value, exercising cognitive control, mentalizing, reasoning, imagining, and interpreting social cues. At the core of moral development are interconnected brain systems responsible for moral emotion, moral reasoning, moral motivation, and moral behavior.

Scientists are revealing that an individual's subjective moral health results from an integration of multiple automatic neural responses that influence behavior. These responses are primarily linked to social emotions and the interpretation of others' actions and intentions. They are beginning to demonstrate that human nature includes an organic moral system. This neural network affects how a person develops behaviors, which either foster or hinder the growth of moral health.

The neuroscience of moral health began with the study of brain damage that causes antisocial behavior. Patients with damage to the ventromedial prefrontal cortex (vmPFC) were found to make poor real-life decisions because they lacked the feelings that guide complex decision-making, as seen in healthy individuals. Researchers discovered that early-onset vmPFC damage led not only to poor judgment but also to a more psychopathic behavioral profile.[40]

Neuroscience reveals that the ventromedial prefrontal cortex (vmPFC) plays a crucial role in encoding the emotional value of sensory stimuli and is significant in emotional processing, which contributes to the generation of

---

[40] Anderson, S W, et.al. Impairment of social and moral behavior related to early damage in human prefrontal cortex. Nature Neuroscience, 2, (1999).

moral emotions.[41] This influences moral motivation, decision-making, and behavior related to a person's moral well-being. This brain region is closely linked to a person's everyday moral skills, reasoning, and behavior.

Only in recent decades have we begun to understand how brain mechanisms can represent a person's moral sense and behavior. We now have a clearer understanding of the limits of moral health based on conventional morality and recognize the differences in moral health levels when someone actively works to improve it. We possess a scientific understanding of the brain mechanisms involved in human thinking, feeling, and motivation, as well as their influence on daily behaviors related to moral health. We understand the difference between simply possessing morality and having moral health.

Neuroscientific researchers have helped us better understand the cognitive and emotional processes behind the origins of everyday behaviors that influence moral health. They demonstrate that behaviors detrimental to moral health are associated with heightened cognitive conflict and shifts in perceptual attention. The brain networks involved in abstract moral judgment and hypothetical decision-making are influenced by fundamental neural mechanisms such as visual perception and reward processing.[42]

Research has been conducted on various human behaviors to uncover the neural basis of actions that influence people's moral health or disease. We will explore what neuroscience shows about brain mechanisms and chemistry in both healthy and unhealthy individuals.

Typically, most people internalize moral norms into their brain's reward system. The habituation of norms happens as a physical process through repeated behavioral training during early years. Neuroimaging studies have shown that one of the most prominent aspects of moral development at the

---

[41] Sommer M, Rothmayr C, et al. How should I decide? The neural correlates of everyday moral reasoning. Neuropsychologia, vol. 48 (2010)

[42] Greene JD. The cognitive neuroscience of moral judgment (2009) in Gazzaniga MS (Ed), The Cognitive Neuroscience (4th ed.), MIT Press

neural level from early childhood to early adolescence is the involvement of brain regions related to motivation and reward systems. In practicing conventional morality, the habituation of norms affects the daily neural mechanisms underlying people's moral behaviors. However, it can also impede the further development of their moral reasoning and moral self.

The early habituation of moral norms leads to behaviors driven by external imperatives. The development of moral capacities from normative morality for moral behavior does not emphasize working towards the greater good, empathetic kindness, interdependence, social responsibility, or the abilities inherent to human nature and what it means to be human. Habituating moral norms overlooks the brain's innate potential to promote moral health through the development of a more mature moral self, higher-order personhood, holistic well-being, and a more meaningful life. These aspects become less significant compared to moral prescriptions, norms, and ideals.

Neuroscience shows that the neural effects of habituation influence the neuroplasticity of brain regions involved in moral behaviors.[43] However, the habituation and internalization of rules develop earlier than the brain regions responsible for advanced cognitive abilities. The brain areas for moral reasoning—which are based on prudence, self-control, and deep self-reflection—mature beyond adolescence. This indicates that higher purposes and ideals grow through self-evolution rather than mere habituation.

Research on altruism and cooperation is key to understanding moral behavior. It has revealed the neural processes involved in developing an other-centered life orientation that motivates people to incur personal costs to help others willingly. Researchers have shown that altruism and cooperation engage

---

[43] Mills KL, et al. Structural brain development between childhood and adulthood: Convergence across four longitudinal samples. Neuroimage. 2016

Merchie, A., & Gomot, M. Habituation, Adaptation and Prediction Processes in Neural Development Disorders: A Comprehensive Review. Brain Sci (7) (2023)

the complex functions of the dorsal insula and amygdala regions of the brain.[44] The value placed on altruism and cooperation, along with the discounting of benefits gained at others' expense, is driven by these brain regions. The research highlights the importance attached to the outcomes of one's actions and behaviors in building moral health.[45]

We live in a world where the moral climate shapes people's daily moral behaviors. We have a global culture that influences everyday thoughts and feelings, significantly shaping people's moral emotions, rationality, and motivation for actions. This culture weakens the purposefulness of the moral self and the importance of developing moral health. Cultural critics argue that this global culture encourages a diminished moral self and moral skills, which can justify people's moral emotions and reasoning, thereby influencing their daily behaviors and affecting their overall moral health.

The neurobiology of moral behavior provides significant insight into how the brain processes sensory perception and moral reasoning, influenced by the socio-cultural factors of our time. Researchers have revealed that social cues, pressures, and cultural influences impact neural mechanisms in everyday life.[46] They emphasize the connection between the social and cultural environment and an individual's moral reasoning in choices and decisions. Evidence shows that when cultural standards and values are prioritized, they become more relevant to the brain mechanisms that determine behavior. It is established that brain mechanisms activated by the social and cultural environment shape behaviors that impact moral health.

Furthermore, researchers have demonstrated that social bias is associated with brain activity patterns related to visual perception, which can

---

[44] Crockett, M. J, et.al. Moral transgressions corrupt neural representations of value. Nature Neuroscience, 20(6) (2017).

[45] Apps M A & Ramnani N. The anterior cingulate gyrus signals the net value of others' rewards. Journal of Neuroscience, 34(18) (2014).

[46] Calabro, R. et. al. Trial-by-trial fluctuations in amygdala activity track motivational enhancement of desirable sensory evidence during perceptual decision-making. Cerebral Cortex, Volume 33, Issue 9, 2023. Oxford University Press.

overshadow brain activity associated with executive control. Studies indicate that when people conform to social and cultural standards and expectations, there are changes in brain activity driven by the effects of visual and sensory perceptions on neurocognitive systems. Social cues, pressures, and cultural influences can shape neural mechanisms to follow a line of moral reasoning, enabling individuals to adapt to situations that may conflict with their motivational choices and decisions, ultimately supporting behaviors that benefit moral well-being.

The social-cultural contexts activate cognitive processes that influence how perception and action are connected in the brain's neural circuits, making certain information more relevant to moral choices and decisions. This explains how individuals can endorse and continue engaging in morally questionable behavior. It highlights the social roots of people's default consciousness, primary neurocognitive mechanisms, and the shaping of their moral identity.

In other words, social context and cultural factors influence brain networks, shaping people's daily cognitive and emotional processes that form the more visible moral self in modern society. Moreover, and more importantly, this powerfully highlights that the brain mechanism of awareness is always necessary to counteract the effects of social and cultural influences on brain functions. Our daily awareness depends on the level of our moral consciousness.

A person's awareness is most important in daily actions. Researchers emphasize that behaviors are complex or problematic because they often happen outside our awareness or conscious control. This also highlights how quickly social factors and cultural contexts influence the way behaviors occur.

Our everyday observations of corruption, fraud, or abuse of power often stop at judging such behaviors as unethical, immoral, or even unthinkable, and condemning them. We tend to assume that everyone knows what is morally "right" rather than morally "wrong" and is free to make choices. However, it is not self-evident that behaviors problematic to moral health are always the result of deliberate decisions. Usually, many of our behaviors are influenced by concerns about moral judgment from others and the fear of social condemnation. Few possess the more developed ability of awareness, particularly self-awareness, which arises from more advanced levels of human consciousness.

Today, neuroscience research also reveals the specific roles of perspective-taking, emotional reactivity, and executive functioning in behaviors that impact people's moral health. The organic moral apparatus not only emphasizes that the moral component is intrinsic to human nature and that moral health is essential to overall health, but also helps us advance new approaches to treating behaviors that negatively impact moral health. This is evident in the cases of violent criminals, sex offenders, kleptomaniacs, pathological liars, and other morally depraved populations, as well as in the evolving criminal justice system.

There is consensus among neuroscientists that emotions play a key role in the cognitive processes that lead to moral motivation, choices, and decisions regarding behavior. The process by which moral emotions operate is believed to be mostly unconscious. Still, the speed at which these emotions enter consciousness suggests they are deeply rooted in the human brain's higher cognitive functions. Neuroscience also reveals that specific neural patterns regulate the level of moral health in individuals, and thus, they can be influenced by the presence of certain neurological disorders.

The understanding of the "moral brain" and its influence on people's behaviors is increasingly impacting how the legal system makes moral judgments. Legal experts emphasize that abnormal behavior resulting from biological anomalies should not render a person morally or legally responsible for problematic actions. The evolving legal perspective on criminal behavior suggests that accountability extends beyond mere violation of the law when it comes to actions that harm moral well-being.

The Clinical Neuroanatomy of Moral Self

The functional and clinical neuroanatomy of moral emotion, moral reasoning, and moral behavior also powerfully demonstrates that a brain network is involved in the development of moral self. The neural functions responsible for fostering moral health also imply the development of the moral self, which is the primary instrument for cultivating moral health. The "moral brain" offers the potential to develop the cognitive and psychoemotional abilities of the moral self. Emotional features that appear in moral reasoning and moral motivation—such as prosocial personality and behaviors—indicate the beneficial aspects of the moral self. Central to the functional moral self for promoting moral health is an individual's self-centered or other-centered orientation and disposition in life.

Research on brain lesion studies focusing on human moral reasoning showed that damage to the prefrontal cortex caused a significant decline in social and moral adjustment.[47] Although the ability to make judgments remained intact for a while, a person's social-moral character traits (moral self) and behaviors rapidly regressed to their state immediately after an accident. Studies examining the link between lesions in the medial prefrontal cortex—which is involved in empathy, motivation, moral reasoning, and related neural processes of the moral self—found that damage to this area during adulthood led to severe social-moral maladjustment and engagement in morally inappropriate behaviors. This suggests that the moral self is deeply intertwined with brain mechanisms.

Understanding the "moral brain" and its behavioral counterpart raises several potentially important clinical issues about people's moral self and their everyday experience of moral health. The "moral brain" is, more or less, the entire brain, using its computational powers for complex psychological and emotional features that are expressed through empathetic amiability, other-

[47] Varrier, RS & Finn ES, Seeing Social: A Neural Signature for Conscious Perception of Social Interactions. The Journal of Neuroscience, Volume 42, Issue 49, 2022

orientedness, compassion, altruism, and similar positive traits of the individual's moral self. These features, or the absence of them, indicate a person's moral capacities as represented by the moral self.

Most people tend to compare themselves to others. They may even downplay their own, often more virtuous, moral self to conform to social and cultural standards and expectations. When individuals modify their worldviews to what they believe is morally acceptable, they may internalize the socio-cultural beliefs, values, and attitudes that shape their moral self, even if it means displaying morally questionable behavior. The structure of the moral self is based on institutional rationality and institutional truth, which social institutions establish.

The researchers noted that when people align their moral self with others, it is because they cognitively engage with appealing social cues and cultural influences, conforming to their socially conditioned moral aptitude and disposition. The research shows that when attention is focused on socially influenced and validated life performances, there is increased activity in the neurocognitive system that affects the neural mechanisms involved in shaping and developing one's moral self. This suggests that social and cultural factors play a significant role in shaping people's moral selves, influencing everyday moral reasoning and moral behavior.

Neuroscience highlights that neural mechanisms are involved in social processes that influence the moral self. Research indicates that when people conform to social and cultural standards and expectations, their brain activity changes due to the effects of visual perceptions on neurocognitive systems.[48] These neural mechanisms use moral reasoning to help individuals adjust if their behavior conflicts with their desired or preferred moral self.

---

[48] Ellemers, N & Nunspeet, F. Neuroscience and the Social Origins of Moral Behavior: How Neural Underpinnings of Social Categorization and Conformity Affect Everyday Moral and Immoral Behavior. Sage Journals (Vol. 29, Issue 29), 2022

The automatic cognitive processes generated by social-cultural contexts undermine and redirect people's intrinsic motivations and intuitions, which usually serve higher-order personhood and the more desired moral self. Neuroscience studies suggest that the motivation for an individual's moral self and behavior results from the affective and rewarding processes of the socio-cultural factors involved in shaping moral views and motivation, typically influencing people's everyday behavior.

Research has shown that the positive bias of social and cultural influences reinforces increased activity in the action-perception neural mechanism. The evidence suggests that individuals are less likely to process information about moral behaviors when their moral self is based on maintaining positive impressions from their social influencers. Additionally, the more motivated individuals are to act, the more vulnerable they become to self-biased views of their moral self. This could explain some of the reasons behind the widespread moral lapses and failures in daily life. These self-biased views are considered self-relevant and serve as the foundation for the individual's moral reasoning. Such moral beliefs lead people to assume that they inherently know what is "morally" right, as opposed to "morally" wrong, and therefore are "morally."

Furthermore, neuroscience studies have examined brain activity related to the reward value of material and social gains. The studies reveal similar patterns of brain activity in the neural mechanisms for both. Researchers show that in the moral domain, people often struggle to reflect on the true origins of their choices, including how these are influenced by others, which they tend to justify after the fact. However, research also indicates that people are not equally affected by the source of social influence and often adapt to more desired influences, positively enhancing their sense of self. This highlights how people are free and deliberate in developing their moral reasoning and behavior, supporting the growth of an individualized moral self.

Neuroscience provides evidence identifying the brain networks involved in the cognitive and affective processes that shape people's daily thoughts, feelings, and behaviors, which reflect the active moral self.[49] On one hand, we understand that morally problematic behaviors are not always deliberate choices. On the other hand, social and cultural contexts can influence the brain mechanisms that create the active moral self of an individual. The evidence suggests that we should not underestimate the impact of social and cultural factors, as well as the self-centered and other-centered orientations and dispositions, on the brain networks involved in cognitive and affective processes that underpin the development of the moral self and the cultivation of moral health.

Generally, people do not assess their moral self to understand their moral reasoning and motivation, which are shaped by social influences. They tend to be less critical of these influences and adopt a moral self molded by the social and cultural environment. They demonstrate moral behaviors aligned with ideals that are socially and culturally conditioned. The highly competitive nature of the world sustains a moral self engaged in morally questionable behaviors rooted deeply in social and cultural factors. The rat race of modern times has diminished the ability to recognize genuine human feelings mentally. We are increasingly unable to experience empathetic and altruistic concerns beyond superficial expressions influenced by social and cultural norms and expectations.

The brain networks of the typical mindset in the postmodern world, influenced by global cultural factors, significantly reduce the neural mechanisms of empathy, altruism, and otherness in people. Cultural stimuli hinder the neural processes that allow a person to be morally critical of social and cultural influences on their moral self. The failure to be the human person one truly is

---

[49] DeYoung, C.G. Personality Neuroscience and the Biology of Traits. Social and Personality Psychology Compass. (Vol 12); 2010
Canli, T. (Ed.) Biology of personality and individual differences. Guilford Press; 2006

and can be results from brain functions and chemistry. This may explain why we encounter people who tend to think that others are less worthy of moral consideration and are more likely to engage in immoral behavior toward them. This tendency is most evident in the use-and-throw culture of our times. Today, it is a common tendency for people to devalue, diminish, and neglect those who may be of no use or no longer helpful.

However, neuroimaging studies reveal the general neural mechanisms behind responsibility and intention in people's behavioral motivation, indicating that external motivations do not entirely drive moral reasoning. These studies have demonstrated that the brain circuitry associated with self-responsibility is significantly activated during moral decision-making tasks and interacts closely with brain regions involved in moral processing.[50]

At the neural level, current research has only measured the connectivity between brain regions involved in moral reasoning within processes like stimulus evaluation, perspective-taking, response selection, empathy, motivation, and similar functions that relate to a person's moral reasoning, moral motivation, and moral behavior, all of which are reflected in the moral self. There are no scientific studies that explore the nature and development of the moral self. However, neuroimaging research consistently shows that the ventromedial prefrontal cortex and orbitofrontal cortex, which are part of the default mode network of selfhood, are also strongly linked to moral reasoning and prosocial behaviors that reflect one's moral self.

There is no scientific knowledge about the structural changes in brain regions associated with the default neural-network mode of selfhood to examine the development of the moral self at the level of brain structure. If there had been, we could compare brain anatomy between ordinary people and the moral paragons, whose distinct moral self is admirably revered. What is certain, however, is that the moral self relying on moral reasoning for behaviors

---

[50] Morris LS, et. al. On what motivates us: a detailed review of intrinsic V. extrinsic motivation. Psychol Med. Volume 52, Issue 10, 2022

is central to one's self-concept. It is also clear that specific brain regions develop moral reasoning, which is reflected in the moral self. Typically, the everyday moral self in people is shaped by brain regions involved in their cognitive and affective abilities.

There is no neuroscientific study directly examining the moral self within a person's self-identity. However, through the proper development of interconnected cognitive and emotional capacities, we can cultivate moral reasoning, motivation, and behavior to foster a self-identity that positively influences moral health. Neuroscience also reveals that the default mode network, which is involved in self-identity, deactivates certain brain regions when individuals engage in cognitive tasks such as self-introspection, which are essential for intentional moral reasoning.[51]

There has been no research on people regarded as moral exemplars and paragons in communities worldwide. The strong functional connectivity of the brain regions in the default network mode for self-identity in moral paragons or exemplars has not been explicitly studied or verified. Since the well-developed moral self of these individuals is integrated with their self-identity, it seems clear that the functional connectivity between brain regions responsible for moral reasoning and the moral self would differ significantly from that of ordinary people. Some experts speculate that the brains of moral exemplars and paragons could be compared to those of ordinary people through reverse-engineering methods.

The Clinical Neuroanatomy of Moral Health and Moral Disease

In our world, the moral health of ordinary people is reflected in the chaos of human life. We see the moral decline of humanity as a serious threat to human existence. Heartless and cold-blooded villains, geopolitical conflicts, brutal community hostilities, and the ongoing inhumane violence—such as large-scale heinous crimes, mass killings, global terrorism, devastating wars, and

---

[51] Davey, CG et.al. Mapping the self in the brain's default mode network. NeuroImage, ScienceDirect, Volume 132, 2016

barbaric genocide—highlight a world in chaos.

The troubling times we live in are also reflected, on no lesser scale, in people's dishonesty, abuse of power and public trust, and corruption and misconduct. We see it in duplicitous individuals, double standards, narcissistic tendencies, hypocritical behaviors, and insatiable greed. All of these are negative signs of our humanity's moral health decline.

Although the neural foundations of the moral health phenomenon are still being studied, neuroscience shows that developing moral health involves multiple overlapping brain circuits rather than a single one. It is established that the operation of neural systems working together to produce moral reasoning, moral emotion, and moral behavior influences moral health. The neurobiological basis of moral health encompasses numerous neural systems and brain mechanisms that influence daily thinking, emotions, motivation, and behavior.

The researchers aimed to identify differences between typical and psychiatric populations.[52] The findings suggest that in healthy individuals, the pain and distress of others serve as a powerful cue, motivating prosocial behaviors aimed at alleviating suffering and condemning harmful actions. They observed that individuals with sociopathy and psychopathy lack moral scruples despite having otherwise intact intellects. This absence manifested as impulsivity, shallow emotional affect, cold indifference, and a lack of guilt and remorse, highlighting their pathological callousness and irresponsibility.

Sociopathy and psychopathy are characterized by an extreme level of callousness, a lack of empathy or emotional depth, and no genuine remorse for harmful behaviors. Psychopathic traits exist on a spectrum that extends into the general population. Psychopaths also tend to be impulsive and have weak emotional responses to harm.

Sociopathy and psychopathy are closely associated with abnormal

---

[52] Neuromorality. Wikipedia Free Encyclopedia.

neuronal activity in specific brain regions and unusual structural connections between them. It primarily results from dysfunction in the amygdala, which is vital for stimulus-reinforcement learning related to socially harmful outcomes and behaviors.[53] The victims of these conditions exhibit significant emotional deficits related to their moral violations. The amygdala, a crucial structure for emotional learning and memory, plays a vital role in this deficiency.

Neuroscience emphasizes that the regions most consistently associated with antisocial behavior are the frontostriatal pathway and/or the amygdala or anterior temporal lobe. The evidence indicates that dysfunction in these neural networks can increase the likelihood of antisocial behaviors. Prosocial behaviors require the swift coordination of multiple neurocognitive systems in brain regions that influence cognition, empathy, and motivation.

Consistent with studies of psychopathology, research on how healthy brains respond to moral transgressions and opportunities emphasizes the importance of the frontostriatal pathway and the amygdalae-vmPFC circuit. It was found that extraordinarily altruistic people tend to have larger amygdalae, which make them more sensitive to feelings and emotions in others.

Research on values and beliefs that influence daily behaviors shows that the temporoparietal junction (TPJ) is the brain area responsible for encoding information about one's beliefs and values.[54] The TPJ is involved in mental states more broadly and is most reliably linked to representing morally relevant mental states. Consistent with this, psychopaths and patients with brain damage in the TJP region exhibit a condition that decreases awareness of their own emotional states, misjudges harm to others as acceptable, and shows reduced emotional responses to harmful outcomes.

It is clear in our society that criminal behavior is often linked to

---

[53] Blair, R.J. The amygdala and ventromedial prefrontal cortex in morality and psychopathy. Trends in Cognitive Sciences, (Vol 11), 2007
[54] Decety J & Cowell JM. Interpersonal harm aversion as a necessary foundation for morality: A developmental neuroscience perspective. Development and Psychopathology, April 2017

psychiatric issues.[55] Violence and crimes indicate that severe mental health conditions can impair moral judgment and motivation. The connection between mental health and moral well-being is an enduring one that has long fascinated philosophers and has become the focus of numerous scientific studies in recent decades.

Neuroscientists have shown that criminal offenders experience significant impairments in parts of the neuro-moral circuit.[56] Dysfunction in the dorsolateral prefrontal cortex has been associated with antisocial traits, including impulsivity and a lack of social inhibition. Problems in the anterior cingulate are associated with reduced emotional processing and increased aggression. Damage to the ventromedial prefrontal cortex has been connected to antisocial behavior, poor and amoral decision-making, and diminished autonomic responses to emotionally charged stimuli. Structural and functional impairments of the amygdala have been observed in psychopathic individuals and criminals, preventing them from recognizing threat signals, making them less fearful and more prone to engaging in antisocial behavior.

Neurological examinations of criminal offenders often reveal significant deficits or changes in the frontal or temporal regions in neuroimaging or electroencephalography. Deficits in frontal functions, such as the inability to adjust responses (response reversal learning) or to inhibit risk-taking behavior after negative feedback, are common among institutionalized and violence-prone individuals. However, some of these deficits might stem from alcohol or substance abuse or other confounding factors, and future research should consider these variables.

It is established that individuals who commit violent crimes often exhibit a high rate of neurological changes. In one study, nearly two-thirds of

---

[55] Decety J & Yoder KJ. Empathy and motivation for justice: Cognitive empathy and concern, but not emotional empathy, predict sensitivity to injustice for others. Social Neuroscience, Vol 11 (2015)

[56] Young, L. et.al. Psychopathy increases perceived moral permissibility of accidents. Journal of Abnormal Psychology, 121(3), (2012).

murderers had neurological diagnoses, including brain injuries, intellectual disability, cerebral palsy, epilepsy, dementia, and other conditions.[57] Researchers have documented evidence that neuroanatomical abnormalities, such as tumors, injuries, or other forms of brain damage, indicate that some criminal defendants may lack the ability to understand right from wrong or to behave according to social norms.[58]

As we discussed earlier, research evidence indicates that the brain structures involved in a person's moral reasoning and behavior are the frontal and temporal cortices, along with specific subcortical structures. The frontal lobe, especially the orbital and ventromedial prefrontal cortices, plays a key role in moral behavior. It is directly involved in emotionally driven decisions, leading to behaviors that can negatively impact a person's moral health. Weak moral emotions and moral rationality diminish moral motivation for actions.

While relying on various underlying cortical areas, an individual's moral sense and moral behavior also depend on a distributed neural network that connects cortical and subcortical structures, modulated by neurotransmitters and hormones. Among subcortical structures, the amygdala is key in processing moral emotions, and when it is damaged or dysfunctional, it can lead to violence. From a behavioral perspective, violence has serious consequences for moral health.

Violence can be defined as any behavior aimed at harming or injuring another person, and when individuals are not motivated to seek treatment, it tends to occur more often. Violence results from multiple factors, including social learning, frustration, cognitive and emotional development, mental and neurological disorders, and environmental and genetic influences. However, some researchers argue that violence is not necessarily caused by brain disease

---

[57] Kiehl KA & Hoffman MB. The criminal psychopath: History, neuroscience, treatment, and economics. Jurimetrics, Vol 51 (2011)

[58] Sterzer, P. Born to be criminal? What to make of early biological risk factors for criminal behavior? Am J Psychiatry, vol. 167 (2010)

or abnormalities in individuals.[59]

Research data on healthy subjects indicate that the frontal lobe governs moral behavior and that different frontal areas likely have distinct roles during moral decision-making. The orbital and ventromedial prefrontal cortices appear to influence moral decisions emotionally. In contrast, the dorsolateral prefrontal cortex mainly functions as a rational 'filter.' This dual process involving the ventromedial prefrontal cortex and the dorsolateral prefrontal cortex appears to be mediated by the anterior cingulate cortex. The amygdala plays a crucial role in processing social and emotional content, particularly in learning that specific actions hurt others and should be avoided. The amygdala seems to be a key subcortical structure involved in processing moral emotions.

Effective diagnosis and treatment are essential for improving health, both in individuals and society. This also encompasses the moral aspect of health, which is an integral part of overall well-being. Understanding the dysfunctional genetic, endocrine, and brain structures that underlie abnormal behaviors affecting moral health can lead to treating pathological aggression, violence, and other forms of immoral behavior—especially when rehabilitation programs fail to produce change.

Recognizing acquired neural abnormalities that affect moral judgment, moral emotions, moral reasoning, and moral behavior raises significant clinical concerns about the moral health of individuals whose choices, decisions, and actions have indelible impacts on others' lives. David Owen described in his book 'In Sickness and in Power' several cases of leaders responsible for states and nations who made critical political decisions while suffering from various neurological conditions.[60] There needs to be an acknowledgment of the moral health issues among those in leadership and authority roles that influence

---

[59] Fabian JM. Neuropsychological and neurological correlates in violent and homicidal offenders: a legal and neuroscience perspective. Aggress Violent Behav, vol.15, (2010)
[60] Owen D. In sickness and in power: illness in heads of government during the last 100 years. Methuen Publishing Ltd (2008)

society and the world.

Many political experts, social and cultural critics, health professionals, and members of the scientific community are increasingly recognizing that the malignant moral self of our time, which is causing a global moral health crisis, is seriously endangering the ideals of life, liberty, and happiness for all. The increasing global issues of crime and violence should be viewed more through the lens of neurological conditions and factors that hinder good moral health. Today, improving moral health requires treatments beyond just rehabilitation programs and invasive neuromodulation techniques. Experts argue that there needs to be more pharmacotherapy to treat and enhance people's moral health.

Human behaviors that lead to violence and criminal acts not only violate standards of morality, ethics, and civil rights but also have serious, unseen effects on mental, physical, and social health.[61] The moral nature of humans is a fundamental element of overall health. Currently, understanding the neural basis of moral health is aiding in the development of new strategies for treating abnormal behaviors such as shoplifting, chronic drug abuse, and serial sexual offenses.

It would be beneficial if scientific knowledge provided the tools to cultivate and develop a moral self that supports the development of moral health. It could accelerate humanity's moral progress and refresh the moral environment of the world if scientific techniques existed to enhance brain regions involved in moral emotions, moral reasoning, and moral behaviors.

However, neuroscience research findings alone are unlikely to help us cultivate and build moral health. It will also require social models to serve as benchmarks of good moral health. Neuroscientists are confident that cultivating and building moral health involves interconnected intellectual abilities such as proper stimulus evaluation, perspective-taking, response selection, empathy, motivation, and self-conception.

---

[61] Baron R. A., & Richardson D. R. Human Aggression. Plenum Press (2004)

Since the beginning of the 21st century, the scientific community has been actively exploring and discussing the neural basis of moral health, just as modern health scientists have been examining other aspects of holistic health. The neural processes and mechanisms involved in cognition, emotion, and behavior are considered crucial to understanding people's moral health. Many agree that the separation between science and moral behavior is an illusion, and potentially dangerous at this point in history. The more we learn about the neuroscience of moral health, the better we can understand what happens when it malfunctions through daily thoughts, feelings, and actions.

HOW TO IMPROVE MORAL HEALTH

Moral health is a crucial component of overall well-being, not merely a metaphor. It relates to the concept of positive health, emphasizing the importance of moral well-being. A person's moral health is vital; healthcare efforts are ineffective without it. Enhancing moral health is a responsibility we owe both to ourselves and to others.

Throughout history, caring for one's health has been a core value of human life. Today, we must more clearly recognize that our primary duty is to promote and maintain good health. Currently, the concept of holistic health extends beyond the traditional physical and mental aspects. It is acknowledged that optimal health is always closely connected to the natural powers of the mind, spirit, and body, working in harmony with the natural world.

The promotion of good health is both a science and an art that involves creating a strong link between one's core passions and all aspects of optimal health. It requires taking responsibility for self-improvement and also includes encouraging the well-being and happiness of others.

People who inspire a more meaningful, noble, and radiant life truly create a "good life' by maintaining high health standards across all areas, cultivating therapeutic relationships, and serving the greater good. However, achieving this requires effort and often involves hardship. They stay grounded in the reality of their present, past, and future, working to preserve what is genuine about human dignity. They intentionally consider the well-being of future generations, just as those before us looked out for ours. They are in a continuous process of growth, striving to become the best version of themselves.

Health literature emphasizes the importance of moral health not only for an individual's well-being but also for society and humanity as a whole. The duty to develop and maintain moral health is mainly outward-facing, meaning it always develops within the context of relationships and real-life situations. The outcomes of our daily choices, decisions, and actions, which impact our moral health, also influence others and the moral well-being of humanity.

Since ancient times, positive ideas about health have included self-governance. For example, promoting health in Plato's philosophy involved cultivating the cardinal virtues: practical wisdom for sound judgment, courage to face dangers, temperance in controlling one's appetites, and demonstrating inner harmony through virtuous behavior. Aristotle introduced the idea of eudaimonia, which means "good spirit," referring to the pursuit of excellence with all one's abilities and dedication. Throughout history, different cultures have employed various methods and techniques to help people develop their self-governing skills in everyday life. Practices such as meditation and yoga remain popular today for self-improvement of the mind, body, and spirit. Self-governance is essential for managing daily health, particularly in terms of its behavioral aspects.

It is a fundamental part of human nature to push past limits and unify the human person, as seen in self-governance. Self-governance essentially involves the influence the moral self has over oneself and is crucial for developing moral health, which ultimately forms the foundation of overall health. A person's moral health depends on their ability to regulate their behavior, which affects all areas of health.

The "good life" involves more than just material wealth. It must include the well-being of the mind, body, and spirit, fostering the "unified" and "whole" human being that one can become. It is about unlocking the full potential of one's humanity. It is rooted in the higher-order personhood that can develop in us high ideals, virtuous character, and meaningful coexistence. Those who uphold human decency, recognize our interdependence, and foster human solidarity demonstrate that these qualities are learned skills accessible to everyone.

The root of toxicity in our global moral environment stems from our behavioral problems. Threats to humanity's future and the planet come from our actions and lifestyle choices. Ongoing discussions focus on the connection between awareness and behavior. Health researchers are particularly interested in what influences people's reasoning and how it shapes their actions. Specifically, they examine whether moral decisions based on reasoning consistently lead to behaviors that impact one's moral well-being.

For a long time, moral behaviors have been judged mainly by verbal and rational views, based on social, cultural, and legal norms—without considering the neurological factors that influence moral reasoning and actions. However, now that neuroscience is combined with findings from psychology and related fields, we can explore the lasting philosophical questions about self-governance, moral conduct, and moral health.

Modern health sciences consider moral health to be more than just acting ethically; they view human consciousness and self-evolution as vital to moral well-being. An evolving consciousness and a morally maturing person influence behavior differently than when actions are based solely on traditional morality. The logic and reasoning behind understanding how behavior affects well-being are more effective than relying only on institutional rationality.

The scientific community is increasingly emphasizing the vital role of behavioral monitoring and management in healthcare. Developing healthy habits and behavioral patterns makes it easier to maintain and improve good health than we often realize. Self-governance generally encompasses the moral aspects of human life, promoting healthy habits and behaviors. Healthy behaviors reduce the risk of poor health conditions and improve how we connect as humans.

Today, the discussion on moral health has highlighted certain risks and misconceptions. Many equate traditional morality with moral health, meaning acting in line with cultural beliefs, values, and norms. It involves living according to these standards. However, in difficult situations and moral dilemmas, individuals often struggle to prioritize correctly the appropriate moral response and behavior. Conflicting responsibilities can lead to actions that don't align with their moral reasoning and motivation to respond relevantly and effectively to moral issues.

Let's examine the health-related challenges stemming from a confused understanding of moral health development, rooted in abstract moral concepts.

Since the Enlightenment, traditional morality has been subject to criticism. Many scholars have strongly spoken out against the harm it causes. Freud and Nietzsche criticized traditional morality as a contributor to poor mental health.[62] Both warned against the excessive guilt, fear, and anxiety that conventional morality can create. Critics argue that traditional morality often overlooks the profound human capacity to experience awe and wonder, unity and love, transcendence and completeness, altruism and gratitude, as well as serenity and peace. Modern health sciences see these experiences as essential for vibrant health, healing, and overall well-being, leading to a better quality of life.

We often rely on traditional morality to judge our self-worth and that of others. Every day, people feel intense guilt and shame for actions that violate these moral standards. This affects other aspects of health without us realizing it. Traditional morality can also prevent people from confronting the real challenges of critical thinking, acting responsibly, and behaving maturely in

---

[62] Freud, S. New Introductory Lectures on Psychoanalysis. W.W.Norton & Company, (1933)
Nietzsche, F. Beyond Good and Evil: Prelude to a Philosophy of the Future. Random House, (1966)

ways that support overall health, especially moral health.

When traditional morality conflicts with deeper insight and sensory perception, people often feel trapped, silently conforming to repetitive and sentimental behaviors. In everyday life, prescriptive morality tends to override people's natural moral instincts. An individual may find it challenging to consider complex, specific circumstances that might require them to act differently than expected. However, moral exemplars demonstrate that moral well-being doesn't rely solely on internalized norms but also on a more nuanced understanding of the present moral situation.

In every moment of a moral dilemma, there is the moral emotion and motivation of the moral sense that are appropriate to it from one's innate moral capacities. It may drive the individual to stray from conventional morality and redirect their actions by reflectively focusing on higher ideals, the greater good, and long-term goals. Often, when building moral health, there may be a need for us to disregard prescriptive morality, cultural norms, and societal laws.

People face daily conflicts between their ideals and convictions, with feelings and actions influenced by traditional morality. They are often hesitant to challenge the outdated thinking patterns that guide moral behavior. The everyday sentimental acts that help them maintain moral norms and ideals usually go unchallenged. Sometimes, this leads people to turn inward and take their own lives. We see reports of suicide driven by guilt and shame among both ordinary individuals and celebrities.

Although our ethical and moral systems provide a solid foundation for prosocial behaviors, they do not always enable us to develop the moral abilities necessary for moral health. Simply adhering to traditional morality does not indicate a person's moral well-being. What stands out in society is that conventional morality often fails to nurture human decency and dignity, or a sense of shared humanity and human solidarity that reflect higher ideals and represent a richer, nobler, and more radiant life.

The common belief is that civil and criminal penalties address moral issues and promote people's moral well-being. However, this is not true in postmodern society! Our legal system can detect and punish violations of the law. Still, it fails to recognize actual signs of moral health, such as higher ideals and purposes in life, higher-order personhood, and psychosocial maturity. It does not help people develop empathy, altruism, cooperation, or a sense of the greater good, nor does it encourage intentional actions toward a healthier humanity. Additionally, the foundations of our civil and criminal laws are based on moral principles from either the Roman or Victorian eras, which are poorly suited to the diverse societies of the postmodern world.

Many view moral health as primarily about not breaking laws and often focus on avoiding detection or exposure. It's clear in everyday life that people make great efforts to avoid public shame and disgrace, but they tend to care less about causing harm to others. This traditional understanding of moral health is rarely questioned and is passed down through generations. Developing moral health is not just about acting in a "moral manner," but about gaining humane abilities to respond effectively and appropriately to urgent moral issues relevant to life.

For many people, it is hard to imagine that, to grow and maintain moral health, sometimes there may be a need to break with conventional morality and societal laws. Developing moral health essentially depends on an individual's sense of self, driven by feelings of "connection and responsibility" toward the immediate needs of others. It involves being true to one's authentic self at all times. It is less about moral ideals and standards and more about the "truth" phenomenon in everyday life.

This has led health experts, researchers, and scientists to stress that moral health involves more than just acting in a "moral manner." For optimal well-being, both tangible and intangible aspects of human nature must work together in harmony. We understand that the healthcare system's exclusive focus on mechanistic diagnosis and pharmacological treatment has long threatened moral health and eudaimonic well-being. It leverages the rich potential of factors such as self-awareness, self-regulation, and self-improvement in the healing process.

The health industry has medicalized problems that are essentially connected to people's moral well-being. Although health professionals may appear impartial about individuals' moral health, the moral aspects of healing and treatment are always present. For example, alcoholism is not just a disease but also stems from the person's choices, decisions, and behaviors. Treating an alcoholic mainly involves moral considerations because the individual is taught self-governance and responsibility. The same is true for other diseases and treatments, which often involve the moral component of health.

The spiritual and moral dimensions are essential to human nature and crucial for a healthy life. However, many people focus only on physical and mental health, often ignoring these key aspects—an oversight common among the pharmaceutical industry, health professionals, and researchers. Without addressing the spiritual and moral, we risk descending into inner chaos and acting without awareness of the true causes of behaviors that lead to poor health.

In a way, moral human nature plays a crucial role in daily healthcare. It has an innate potential to heal and improve health. Scientific evidence shows the neural basis of moral health, revealing neurobiological factors that support healing and well-being. Nature provides us with the ability to heal through self-governance, which helps us build and maintain moral health.

Growing moral health is closely linked to a person's life orientation, which can be either self-focused or other-focused. In health literature, experts indicate that healthier individuals tend to be more other-oriented. Achieving optimal health depends on a strong moral motivation to connect with the web of life. People who feel deeply connected and interdependent share a sense of responsibility for humanity. They demonstrate a way of being in the world and adopt lifestyles that can improve personal health just as effectively as other methods used to enhance physical and mental well-being.

Neuroscience research shows that people with self-focused traits do not activate the neural circuits usually triggered by other-focused traits.[63] It is recognized that when the neurocognitive systems involved in engaging people in inhibitory control tasks weaken, individuals are also more likely to exhibit weaker moral reasoning and become overconfident, which can compromise moral behavior. Neuroscience highlights that self-focused traits lead to a broad decrease in the functional connectivity between the neurocognitive systems that support a person's moral health.

Today, a clearer understanding of health is emerging: healthy individuals are recognized for demonstrating moral qualities such as compassion, respect, tolerance, integrity, autonomy, social responsibility, high-mindedness, and similar traits. All of these emphasize that an other-centered mindset is crucial for enhancing overall health.

In summary, positive views of health consistently highlight self-governance and assume the moral nature of humans. These moral capacities provide people with their life purpose and meaning in a way that differs from cultural influence. Developing and enhancing one's moral health always involves others in life. An other-focused mindset in thinking, feeling, and actions is essential for cultivating and sustaining moral health.

There are two practical ways to improve moral health. These are (1) addressing cultural factors and influences that weaken the moral self and focusing on developing moral health, and (2) unlocking the full potential of one's humanity.

Addressing cultural factors and influences:

Forces like materialism, consumerism, and individualism shape today's global culture. The destructive spread of individualism and materialism is like a relentless cancer, preventing us from looking beyond the confines of hedonistic

---

[63] Hauser MD. Moral Minds: How Nature Designed our Universal Sense of right and Wrong. Ecco/Harper Collins; 2006

living. We inhale and exhale toxins from a social and cultural environment devoid of higher purpose.

Every day, we must navigate a human existence that is undeniably driven by utilitarianism. It is full of deceit, manipulation, and an insatiable thirst for wealth, fame, and power. We constantly have to manage relentless cultural stimuli designed to trigger biases that support utilitarian thinking. It is the most prominent modern mindset that reinforces attitudes and values that hinder self-awareness, self-evaluation, and self-regulation.

In our self-centered world, we are captivated by illusions about human life and the world, yet at the same time, we have lost our grasp on the reality of who we truly are and what is genuine about the world we inhabit. We have become like puppets engaging only with an illusory life, which we find thrilling and entertaining. We remain indifferent to the moral toxicity and decadence around us. We find ways to silence both the dissenting inner voices within us and the wiser voices from those around us, as Plato observed in 'The Republic,' everything that deceives also charms.

Nevertheless, the moral sense in people remains a basic human desire. It is demonstrated positively through the recovery of addicts and the rehabilitation of criminals. The efforts of non-starters and delinquents toward a "better me" reflect this. Negatively, it is linked to the physical and mental health problems filling hospitals and prisons, the startling statistical evidence of the rise in violent acts and heinous crimes in society, and many other behaviors seen in today's world that harm good healthcare.

In today's world, almost everyone struggles in many ways to overcome the feeling of a soulless, shallow, and empty life. At its core, all our human struggles stem from the moral realm of life. As humans, we experience within ourselves the advanced stage of a morally corrupt self. Daily experiences show us that the reality of a morally corrupt self exists as a spectrum within the general population.

Growing moral health in the postmodern era is often challenging when subconscious cultural scripts and a degraded moral climate make it difficult to distinguish truth from fiction and reality from fantasy. Today, people worldwide face overwhelming mental, emotional, and volitional struggles caused by their social and cultural surroundings. Greed, egotism, and hedonism have overshadowed practical wisdom, moral responsibility, and other-centered life values. These lower instincts threaten not only higher ideals and life purposes but also common sense in everyday life.

Moral health depends on free-choice behaviors and is embedded in the same cause-and-effect framework as the rest of nature. Many factors shape human behavior, but two are especially important for health: self-regulation and habit. Self-regulation is the ability to guide behaviors and control impulses to meet standards, reach goals, and uphold values in life. Habits are behaviors that recur when prompted by specific situations, occur unconsciously, and are learned through repetition.

When human behavior is simplified to habits, it comes from automatic reactions to stimuli. With self-regulation, we act in ways that serve our short and long-term best interests and align with our core values. Habits keep us doing what we've always done, but we need self-regulation to act correctly and appropriately.

Another challenge of postmodern culture is that we see cultural ideas, beliefs, and lifestyles as final. Every day, people unknowingly believe what they are told about their identity through cultural advertisements and social models. Global culture has led ordinary people to pursue human life with increasingly slavish conformity to the world's expectations and demands. We mindlessly conform to and accept cultural standards and values, acting more like actors on a stage, unaware of our true selves or what life is really about.

Our society is obsessed with social status, celebrity fame, and raw power. Our media is filled with unscrupulous characters, hypocrites, and sociopaths whom we imitate. Consumerism urges us toward extravagance by telling us that what we have can never be enough. Materialism leads us to believe that our identity depends on what we possess. We develop attitudes and values that prioritize outward appearance over the inner self. This leaves little room and energy to understand the more profound truths about who we are.

This leads people to make positive, but often incorrect, generalizations about themselves. Naturally, the goal is self-serving. Most remain unaware of their true selves and the reasons behind their behavior. Worse still, many seem satisfied with this state of personal ignorance; they don't believe there's anything more to discover or accomplish. They are indifferent to their moral sense or whatever moral compass they have. This mainly happens because people want to fit in, regardless of the impact on their moral self-integrity and moral well-being. The pitiful consequence is that people become accustomed to hiding their real selves as a means of being themselves, surviving in society with a pseudo-self.

Self-concealment runs so deep that a person rarely recognizes it even in themselves. It is common to boost self-worth and gain personal power through a fake identity. While self-acceptance is valued, an insatiable desire for ego gratification often links it to a false version of oneself. No one – including the individual — truly knows what they are like inside. Deception, cheating, and hypocrisy are often accepted as means to achieve this.

Like glistening black beetles, society's deceptions and untruths crawl into a person's sense of self, giving the individual daily illusions of power and prestige. This mirage of false realities fills an ordinary person's life, trapping them further in the prison of self-flattery and self-centeredness. The individual spins around the axis of the delusional self, unaware that their true self is constantly breaking apart. Yet, this self-disintegration is never seen as a problem. Instead, it makes people seem like they have a multi-layered personality, with inconsistent identities and self-delusions.

Furthermore, each day's routine life gradually consumes all of a person's time, overshadowing any self-awareness and self-evaluation. The global culture of our era avoids introspection, vulnerability, and shared humanity. Most of the time, we can't even picture a better version of ourselves. Living a double life has become commonplace. It's easy to pretend to be someone we're not. Having multiple and even conflicting self-identities is rarely viewed as a moral health issue. When self-delusions and social-cultural forces destabilize a person's sense of self, the individual can't step back enough to explore, evaluate, and regulate themselves.

Research literature shows that self-bias leads people to overestimate themselves, sometimes even creating false evidence to support this view. It also indicates that individuals tend to perceive themselves less accurately than they perceive others. Studies reveal that even when inappropriate self-presentation triggers feelings of guilt, self-doubt, and anxiety, neither the person nor observers can distinguish what is genuine within them.[64] Nowadays, projecting a false, inconsistent self-identity driven by external motives and aimed solely at impressing, persuading, and manipulating others for personal gain has become increasingly common. It has become customary to adopt a confused and evasive self-image that lacks self-truth, the genuine self, and human virtues.

People have become so used to deception and manipulation—both their own and others'—that their entire moral self has become numb. This is evident in a shallow human existence where pretenses, recklessness, and cleverness replace genuine human decency, character, and integrity. It results in people even becoming oblivious to the constant, more profound desire for self-improvement and personal growth. Today, we feel an intense hunger for the freedom of the human spirit. People's stories of a transformed life show that actual change can only happen through moral renewal.

The cycle of self-deception and self-centeredness blocks individuals from developing higher-order thinking. That cycle also stops them from uncovering the false beliefs that constantly fill unsettling mental gaps. Instead of confronting their yet-to-be-known self-truths, people fill any void with more

---

[64] Metzinger, T. The Ego Tunnel: The Science of the Mind and the Myth of the Self. Basic Books (2010)

cultural illusions, reinforcing their self-delusions and risking even more unpredictable consequences.

Self-exploration and self-understanding are crucial parts of how the human mind works. However, today's distorted mindset makes it more difficult for people to distinguish between reality and fantasy. It is a mindset that relies on deception and manipulation to energize individuals. This is evident in the evil actions of our times, where the human consciousness, which includes higher-order thinking, has diminished or leaked out of the human person.

The most brutal battle to fight each day is staying aware of the relentless pressure of social and cultural conformity. Without awareness, we fall victim to an unending toxic moral environment. Focusing on developing moral health appears to be the best and most effective way to become aware of these social and cultural pressures. However, maintaining attention on moral well-being and a better quality of human life appears to become increasingly challenging every day. In general, personal health seems to be only priced when lost. People only begin to focus on developing moral health by confronting who they genuinely are and who they want to be. They realize that there is always a need to reclaim the human dignity they deserve. Self-awareness, then, becomes the path to moral clarity and self-regulation of behaviors.

People with poorly developed self-awareness and critical-thinking skills miss social and cultural cues and fail to process the overwhelming information around them. They are similar to those suffering from anoxia, brain injury, or stroke. They can only operate automatically, not intentionally. They are unable to shift gears to incorporate higher-order thinking, which is essential for adapting to new situations or conditions they face.

Neuroscience research has significantly enhanced our understanding of how neural network processes influence people's everyday feelings, reasoning, and behavior, with profound implications for mental health and moral well-being.[65] The integrity of these processes is the core foundation of an individual's moral self. Evidence shows that dysfunction in these networks can lead to a tendency toward negative behaviors that harm moral well-being.

Neuroscientific evidence suggests that the value we assign to social and cultural stimuli forms the basis of our brain's cognitive and emotional systems, with which we navigate life.[66] These brain systems tend to predispose us toward self-centered orientations. Additionally, cognitive scientists suggest that social and cultural stimuli automatically trigger behaviors deeply rooted in the unconscious.[67] As a result, neurocognitive processes involved in moral reasoning often surpass established conventions and moral norms. We develop moral skills and motivation that lead to a more permissive moral understanding and a constantly evolving moral rationality.[68]

Self-awareness and self-regulation characterize a person's progression in human consciousness, utilizing significant brain energy for growth. The evolving sense of self guides the individual's more profound understanding of daily choices and decisions. In contrast, a person who lacks self-awareness often feels stuck in their comfort zone, indifferent to self-transcendental ideals, high-minded principles, the common good, and character traits such as honesty, integrity, and empathy. Without a solid epistemic foundation on life orientation, values, and goals, they have only a fragmented sense of self and no real power to achieve what they vaguely desire.

People who lack self-awareness have little clarity about who they truly are. They show a superficial self-identity that is inconsistent or only adopted in specific situations. This has become so common that, in today's moral climate, a tragic sense of selfhood is no longer surprising. When chaotic individuals live

---

[65] Sadler-Smth, E. Biology, Brain, Behavior, and the "Moral Sense." Cambridge University Press,(2015)

[66] Raine, A & Yang, Y. Neural foundations to moral reasoning and antisocial behavior. Journal of Social Cognitive and Affective Neuroscience (Vol 1) (2006)

[67] Festinger, L. A Theory of Cognitive Dissonance. Stanford University Press, (1962)

[68] Moll J & de Oliveira-Souza R. Moral judgments, emotions and the utilitarian brain. Trends Cogn Sci. 2007

in a disorderly world without self-awareness and self-understanding, they develop a rotten human psyche that reveals a wretched human condition.

In contrast, when people understand who they are and commit themselves to growing toward their better selves, self-transformation becomes possible. Moral health becomes their primary focus and steadfast goal. They strive for full human potential, like virtuous heroes who embody a high-minded, noble, and radiant life. The life goals of many such individuals often oppose social and cultural influences.

Unlocking the full potential of one's humanity

In his book 'The Moral Animal: Evolutionary Psychology and Everyday Life', Robert Wright writes, "Human beings are a species splendid in their array of moral equipment, tragic in their propensity to misuse it, and pathetic in their constitutional ignorance of the misuse."[69] Despite deep dissatisfaction with a chaotic and messy life, people fervently avoid self-awareness, self-evaluation, and self-development. Personal growth inevitably requires hard work, pain, and deliberate investment of time and energy. Today, by rejecting this effort as too costly, we are betraying the deformity of a moral self for an all-around, holistic human person.

All species evolve by navigating and surviving in their environment. For humans, this is a lifelong process of trial and error, discovery, and learning. It relies on consciousness, which is fundamental to being human. An individual's sense of selfhood is a given reality; it isn't fleeting or an artificial construct. However, because of consciousness, it is not permanent or unchanging.

Consciousness is what makes us self-aware and form a unified whole. It is fundamental to human metaphysical nature. Consciousness is the primary tool we must develop to support self-transcendent ideals. It is the innate ability humans possess to direct thoughts, regulate impulses, and pursue overarching

---

[69] Wright, R. The Moral Animal: Evolutionary Psychology and Everyday Life. Vintage Books (1995)

goals. The capacity for human interrelation and interconnectedness is rooted in consciousness. The individual's experience of human consciousness is deeply felt through the sense of a "whole" self.

Consciousness creates a person's selfhood, the sense of "I." The identity one develops is more than just the influences of human biology, psychology, and the social environment. It involves the metaphysical human tendency to distinguish between the self that is "I" and "not-I." Since the sense of "I" is tied to consciousness, it is constantly modified as a person grows and changes. This often makes a person's sense of selfhood seem ambiguous and quite fluid. Because of this, one's selfhood can seem as elusive as consciousness; it cannot be understood apart from the environment in which one lives.

The universal question, "Who am I?" is a timeless one. Essentially, it is a metaphysical question. It inquires about the profound inner self that lies beneath all a person's thoughts, feelings, behaviors, and experiences.

Metaphysical human nature underpins our self-identity and self-understanding. It is through the ontological reality of selfhood that we interpret, monitor, and govern how we think, feel, and behave in daily life. Today, the concept of this metaphysical self remains just as significant to modern science and technology as it was in ancient philosophy.

The journey toward moral health is ongoing and continually involves the self-evolution of the human person through the evolution of consciousness. Moral health develops when a person's behaviors align with their deepest core and higher aspirations. Cultivating moral health requires self-awareness and self-regulation. In daily life, this means rewiring one's brain to break habits that have become dysfunctional. This only happens when we evolve toward higher levels of human consciousness.

Our values, attitudes, judgments, and behaviors typically evolve, for better or worse, depending on the level of human consciousness. Without the development of consciousness, people have a poor understanding of who they are and what they want to become in life. Consciousness evolution is a neurobiological process, not just an abstract theory of selfhood. There is a need for the brain's mechanisms supporting higher cognitive functions to grow in self-awareness and self-regulation.[70] With deeper self-knowledge derived from sensory perception and intuition, individuals develop a more refined moral self than one shaped solely by conventional morality.

The moral content in the evolving human consciousness, known as moral consciousness, overcomes cultural conditioning and the flawed moral climate of the world. High levels of moral consciousness develop a greater capacity for moral emotion, reasoning, motivation, and behavior, fostering moral well-being. Such levels also remove superficial self-projections and self-centered life views. The increased connectivity between neurocognitive systems responsible for empathetic concern and amiability creates higher-level thinking and a more other-oriented attitude.

When we have a lasting commitment to moral health, we can evaluate who we truly are more accurately and develop into higher forms of personhood. Our way of being in the world is reflected in high levels of personal integrity, an unshakeable character, a mature moral self, and psychosocial maturity.

Every person acts based on a self-definition that influences every part of their life. Most people operate from a self-definition that may be more or less conscious. The self-definition a person uses interacts with their current life situation and social environment, ultimately affecting their overall life.

An individual's self-definition can stem from either a fixed mindset or a growth mindset. Stanford University psychologist and researcher Carol Dweck emphasizes that these two mindsets, which we develop from a very early age, significantly influence our behavior, our relationship with success and failure in both professional and personal contexts, and ultimately our capacity for happiness.[71]

---

[70] Perlovsky, LI & Kozma R (Editors). Neurodynamics of Higher-Level Cognition and Consciousness. Springer-Verlag, (2007)
[71] Dweck, C. Mindset: The New Psychology of Success. Random House (2007)

Someone with a "fixed mindset" views their personality and character as unchanging and permanent. The person values social acceptance and public recognition, aiming for success and avoiding mistakes at all costs. In contrast, a person with a "growth mindset" welcomes challenges and does not see failure as a sign of a character flaw but as an opportunity for growth.

The fixed mindset prevents learning anything new about oneself. People with a fixed mindset tend to easily tolerate ambiguity and inconsistency as they transition from one situation to another. The motives and actions of such individuals are often unclear. Without a sense of a unified self, this incoherence does not bother them. They ignore the signals triggered by the mismatches between feelings, thoughts, attitudes, and behaviors. They fail to protect the integrity of their selfhood from recurring failures to face reality and tend to surrender to fate. These individuals appear disconnected from the actual reality of self and environment. When this occurs, the person inevitably feels disintegrated despite their desperate efforts to hold themselves together. They are only held together by a fundamental desire for self-preservation.

On the other hand, people with a growth mindset always strive for self-awareness and self-improvement. Instead of trying to hide or protect their fragile ego, individuals with a growth mindset see themselves as a dynamic and active process. These self-aware individuals make rational choices for responsible living. The hallmark of people with a growth mindset is that they continually develop their moral capacities and progress in moral health. They aim to be present-oriented, uphold high ideals, grow in other-oriented ways, and build integrity and character by stretching the limits of their psycho-moral abilities. Above all, they overcome hurdles to evolve in their moral self. They enjoy a beneficial increase in moral capacity that enhances well-being and happiness. Such individuals experience an improved sense of wholeness, reflected in a holistic life, enduring happiness, and high levels of moral health.

Today, the numerous enticing options make it challenging to discern what truly benefits a person, especially when their sense of self is weak or uncertain. Environmental triggers are difficult to ignore, and few people take the time to carefully examine the causes and consequences of their decisions and actions. The world presents many 'success' traps that we rarely question. Deceptions, illusions, and tricks are more convincing to those without a strong sense of self.

A fixed mindset means that social and cultural influences can impact every aspect of a person's well-being and happiness. When people are influenced by their social and cultural environment, they often avoid critical thinking about themselves. The pull of their social and cultural world is stronger than the desire for higher goals or inspiration from moral role models who demonstrate virtuous living. If they are unwilling or unable to question their own hypocrisy and double standards, they tend to cling to a false sense of self. In each moment, a fictional idea of who they are guides their actions. When someone's sense of self is unstable, it confuses their identity and how they present themselves to others.

In contrast, a person who adopts a growth mindset looks inward to explore their true self and directs their efforts toward self-improvement to achieve the maturity and wholeness they desire and intend. This growth mindset is founded on the belief that one's self-definition develops in harmony with the evolving moral self and can be cultivated through effort. Although a character flaw may exist, one believes that change and growth are possible through effort and experience. A person with a growth mindset is continually and intentionally challenged to improve their sense of self. With nothing to hide, the individual isn't easily discouraged or overwhelmed by failures. At the core of a growth mindset is a passion for learning rather than seeking approval.

The research highlights the key difference between the two mindsets: for those with a growth mindset, personal success means working the hardest to become their best, while for those with a fixed mindset, success is about establishing superiority, plain and simple.[72] For the latter, setbacks are seen as a verdict and a label on self-identity. For the former, setbacks serve as a wake-up call to motivate change and growth.

Subconsciously, people often assume that public opinion about them is more significant than their actual experiential self-reality. They are driven to protect their public image at all costs, which can easily result in dishonesty, corruption, and hypocrisy. Ironically, this focus on self-preservation fosters an unsettling sense of identity and diminishes moral capacity. When a person filters their sense of self through the social environment, their self-definition becomes vague and disturbing. When people are not working toward wholeness, the natural result is a fragmented sense of self.

How a person views and inhabits the world shapes their response to its demands. Every life situation requires us to stay alert and fully aware of our responses, which can either help us succeed or cause us to fail as humans. When people focus on their daily internal monologues about different aspects of life, they can imagine countless possibilities for personal growth.

There's nothing automatic or inevitable about self-improvement and personal growth. No quick fix or secret method exists in the therapies popularized by culture. An individual's true potential for growth and happiness remains unknown or impossible to predict until they are in the moment, passionately working toward heroic success. Every person can achieve anything related to moral development when their efforts are rooted in a rigorous pursuit of higher-level personhood, which is crucial for growing moral health.

Self-transformation and human growth demand more than just opinions about human decency or high-mindedness. They require the individual's realization that once health, relationships, and dignity are lost, the past cannot be undone. There is an understanding that the journey of self-

---

[72] Dweck C. Mindset – Updated Edition: Changing The Way You Think To Fulfill Your Potential. Little, Brown Book Group, (2017)

transformation is never complete but always progressing toward completion. It may happen gradually, but unless people intentionally pursue it, many may reach old age with nothing but regrets.

A person focused on building moral health engages in objective truth-seeking. They are willing to question any hypocrisy, prejudices, or double standards in their life. All the information they process is positively influenced by the pursuit of the absolute good, the absolute right, and the absolute just course in life. Of course, no one can realistically hope to reach these absolutes, but everyone can aim to keep moving toward them rather than further away. One's mental attitude can have a profoundly positive impact on actions and behavior. They are capable of continually examining their choices and actions to see how well they align with their ultimate intentions.

Typically, growth happens gradually and is often barely noticeable; a person only slowly moves closer to the truth about themselves. Sometimes, there are fleeting yet potentially life-changing "self-truth moments." These moments might be triggered when someone feels shame in public. Or, unexpectedly, a person may suddenly become aware of the gap between who they are and who they pretend to be. Clearly seeing the destructive impact of a fractured sense of self, the person may use this "moral health check-up" as an opportunity to take a significant step toward becoming who they truly want to be.

People who follow this path typically rely on the insights, intuitions, instincts, and perceptions associated with a growth mindset. Moral heroes operate from this growth mindset. Instead of giving up when faced with problems and challenges, they persist with resilience. Because they aren't standing on shaky ground of self-doubt and hesitation, they display herculean strength and push themselves to reach their full human potential. Instead of settling for meeting the world's minimal standards, they tune into the insights of their higher self and gravitate toward higher-order personhood. They become better at detecting and rejecting cover-ups, gimmicks, and superficial societal expectations.

This growth mindset isn't limited to superheroes. Anyone can strive to improve their moral health every day. Every reflective individual deeply yearns to leave the arid wasteland of self-delusions and ego-centricism and journey toward a more meaningful human existence. It begins with the truth of one's unique inner self, the real self, and the inkling into the better version of oneself, but reaches forward toward a self-identity that serves healing purposes. It is shaped by countless moments of inspiration and insight throughout a person's lifetime, leading to a brighter future. The active work on the project of self-transformation serves as an inspiration to others of everything positive in the human experience. It aims at acquiring benefits not only for oneself but also for others. It becomes the individual's silent service and efforts at the renaissance of a better humanity.

The growth mindset is self-validating. In moments of confronting a self-definition shaped by untruths, people realize that there is ongoing self-disintegration, which blocks growth in wholeness and integrity. By facing the inconsistency in their self-identity and selfhood, they intentionally adopt a growth mindset to develop a self that includes moral capacities deliberately. This process demands significant time and effort, but only some are willing to undergo rebirth, nurturing within themselves the brightness of a flame and the fragrance of a flower. They become heroes who aim to leave a virtuous legacy of a noble and radiant life.

Conventional morality depends on people's neural development of habituation and the fixed mindset, rather than on more advanced cognitive skills like the growth mindset. Neuroscience links neural mechanisms of prudence, self-control, empathy, and self-awareness with the more developed and sophisticated moral capacities. Research provides evidence of behaviors judged morally right that do not stem from early habituation or the internalization of moral norms.[73]

Moral health cannot be improved with pills, brain stimulation techniques, or methods that amplify moral thinking, feelings, and behavior, or any other newfangled ideas. Sociological and psychological studies have shown that increasing moral health is strongly influenced by the emulation of historical and long-distance moral role models, as well as the moral exemplars of peers and community members. Additionally, neuroscience studies suggest that enhancing moral health in individuals can be as straightforward as disrupting the neural circuits established during childhood and adolescence for moral reasoning.[74]

---

[73] Walker, LJ. Moral Motivation through the perspective of exemplarity. In Handbook of moral motivation: theories, models, and application, Ed Heinrichs, FO & Lovat T. Sense Publishers (2013)
[74] Harenski, CL., et.al. Neural development of mentalizing in moral judgement from adolescence to adulthood. Dev Cogn Neurosci (1) (2012).

CONCLUSION

The noblest work of anyone's life is to take on the stewardship of one's health, especially moral health, as it involves the ongoing rebirth of one's holistic self. An individual's true potential for self-improvement is unpredictable until one passionately works toward ideals and goals, inspired by the virtuous heroes of a noble and shining life. Even one person's dedication to personal moral health and the moral health of humanity can make it easier for others to envision and achieve the rejection of the empty, desolate human spirit of our age.

Someone who listens to their internal monologues reflects on the harmful effects of the global moral climate on the human spirit, which is marked by chaos and discontentment. There will be moments of awakening to one's self-deceptions and superficial existence. When people start to see who they truly are, they can begin to understand how many problems they have created for themselves and others. This awareness allows people to develop a new belief system that values human authenticity—being open and vulnerable—and promotes humane values and abilities.

A person who focuses on moral health will demonstrate higher-level personhood, psychosocial maturity, and display human virtues such as honor, authenticity, reliability, and compassion. There is alignment between a person's true self and how they present their self-identity to the world. Integrity and character act like the framework of a building. They are vital to a person's self-definition and self-identity. The Latin root of the word integrity suggests wholeness, representing a complete person. Character, widely regarded as the crown of life, is the inner structure that allows one to attain the full measure of selfhood.

However, as people change and grow, success and failure in a person's life will remain binary traps that challenge their moral development and progress. Neither success nor failure is complete or absolute. This fact reminds us to always aim for the ideal, building on successes and learning from failures. Moving toward the ideal is possible; achieving perfection is not. Becoming more moral, healthier, and more whole is achievable.

The pursuit of self-evolution for a stable self-identity is worthwhile. In turn, personal integrity and character will stand firmly above what society superficially deems conventional and acceptable. Such an individual exhibits a selfhood rooted in psycho-moral and psychosocial clarity, not in a robotic self based on socio-cultural influences. Character and integrity remain steadfast. Self-identity represents a whole person, unthreatened by secrets in the closet. What is polite and proper is less critical, but what is noble and radiant is. The individual's vibrant human spirit effectively inspires others to seek self-transformation. They catch a glimpse of a previously unimagined self-identity rich in honor and self-respect. This, in turn, motivates them to develop an individualized moral self, unlike the socially conforming one, which is standardized and preoccupied with conventional morality.

Personal transformation is always intertwined with the transformation of society, culture, and the world as a whole. As individuals shed self-centered protectionism and move toward wholeness, they increasingly realize that they are part of the web of life. One cannot separate personal well-being from global welfare. Human life becomes more meaningful only within the reality of interrelatedness and interconnectedness. The person's attitude shifts from being competitive to collaborative. They treat others with sensitivity, reciprocity, and respect. Instead of deceitfully manipulating others, they embody fairness, empathy, and altruism.

The renewal of the human spirit is the only way humanity's future can be saved. Individuals who become stewards of moral health leave a lasting legacy in the spirit of humanity. In a world we inhabit that is shackled by greed, prestige, and domination, where self-deception is the ultimate coping mechanism of human frailty, everything depends on the stewards of moral health. Though the steps taken will be small, the effort to achieve that stewardship will be enormous. The courageous and exemplary efforts will inspire others to exert the effort they need to develop their moral capacities and embark on the path of virtuous living through a well-developed moral self, cultivated by moral consciousness. More and more people will begin to walk the long and difficult tightrope of hope, aiming not just to survive but to thrive in pursuit of one's whole humanity.

As more people start to weave the cohesive threads that form the web of life, they will share their dreams and noble ambitions. Together, they will daily challenge the shadows that seek to weaken the human spirit. The world won't give up its tricks and gimmicks designed to keep people swelling in all forms of moral disease. The human-robot illusion may cause fear when people open their hearts to rebirth and self-discovery. The old and new struggle fiercely. The old is familiar, and the latest may seem like fiction. Still, renewing the human spirit is possible if people correctly interpret the signs of the times through daily life experiences and their evolving moral awareness. Otherwise, the harmful influence of those with poor moral health will inevitably threaten humanity and the planet.

www.ingramcontent.com/pod-product-compliance
Lightning Source LLC
Chambersburg PA
CBHW060242030426
42335CB00014B/1571